Emergency Guide
for Dental Auxiliaries

FOURTH EDITION

Emergency Guide
for Dental Auxiliaries

FOURTH EDITION

Debra Jennings, D.M.D. / Janet Bridger Chernega

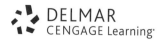

DELMAR
CENGAGE Learning®

Australia • Brazil • Japan • Korea • Mexico • Singapore • Spain • United Kingdom • United States

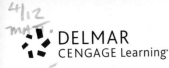

(handwritten notes in top left margin: "4/12 mat" and "a 84.95")

DELMAR CENGAGE Learning·

**Emergency Guide for Dental Auxiliaries,
fourth edition**
Debra Jennings, DMD
Janet Bridger Chernega

Vice President, Editorial: Dave Garza

Director of Learning Solutions:
  Matthew Kane

Senior Acquisitions Editor: Tari Broderick

Managing Editor: Marah Bellegarde

Associate Product Manager: Meghan E. Orvis

Editorial Assistant: Nicole Manikas

Vice President, Marketing: Jennifer Baker

Marketing Director: Wendy Mapstone

Associate Marketing Manager: Scott Chrysler

Production Manager: Andrew Crouth

Content Project Manager: Brooke
  Greenhouse

Senior Art Director: Jack Pendleton

For product information and technology assistance, contact us at
Cengage Learning Customer & Sales Support, 1-800-354-9706

For permission to use material from this text or product,
submit all requests online at **www.cengage.com/permissions**.
Further permissions questions can be e-mailed to
permissionrequest@cengage.com

Library of Congress Control Number: 2012931210

ISBN-13: 978-1-111-13860-8

ISBN-10: 1-111-13860-5

Delmar
5 Maxwell Drive
Clifton Park, NY 12065-2919
USA

Cengage Learning is a leading provider of customized learning solutions with office locations around the globe, including Singapore, the United Kingdom, Australia, Mexico, Brazil, and Japan. Locate your local office at:
international.cengage.com/region

Cengage Learning products are represented in Canada by Nelson Education, Ltd.

To learn more about Delmar, visit **www.cengage.com/delmar**
Purchase any of our products at your local college store or at our preferred online store **www.cengagebrain.com**

Notice to the Reader
Publisher does not warrant or guarantee any of the products described herein or perform any independent analysis in connection with any of the product information contained herein. Publisher does not assume, and expressly disclaims, any obligation to obtain and include information other than that provided to it by the manufacturer. The reader is expressly warned to consider and adopt all safety precautions that might be indicated by the activities described herein and to avoid all potential hazards. By following the instructions contained herein, the reader willingly assumes all risks in connection with such instructions. The publisher makes no representations or warranties of any kind, including but not limited to, the warranties of fitness for particular purpose or merchantability, nor are any such representations implied with respect to the material set forth herein, and the publisher takes no responsibility with respect to such material. The publisher shall not be liable for any special, consequential, or exemplary damages resulting, in whole or part, from the readers' use of, or reliance upon, this material.

Printed in the United States of America
1 2 3 4 5 6 7 17 16 15 14 13 12

Contents

SECTION II   Altered Consciousness Emergencies

41

Chapter 4   Syncope

43

Chapter 5   Seizure Disorders

55

Chapter 6   Diabetes Mellitus

69

Preface

Introduction

Medical emergencies can and do occur within the dental office environment. A large percentage of these emergencies could be prevented or at least better treated if all the members of the dental team were more knowledgeable in the prevention and management of emergency situations.

The *Emergency Guide for Dental Auxiliaries* is designed to provide dental auxiliary students with the basic skills and knowledge necessary in order to function effectively as a member of the dental team. This text is also an effective refresher tool for dental auxiliaries who are already working in dentistry. The format of this textbook will help the reader master new information and will simplify review of previously learned materials.

Why I Wrote This Text

I have used this textbook since the beginning of my teaching career. It contains basic information and a format that allows the educator to use the content as written or increase the knowledge base as appropriate for the level of the students. Because of changes in the standards for CPR, as well as new terminology and teaching modalities, I felt that a new edition would enhance the usability of this textbook as a teaching tool.

Chapter Organization

The fourth edition of *Emergency Guide for the Dental Auxiliary* has seen a tremendous overhaul in the organization and presentation of the chapters. The new layout and order is a result of listening to our customers and designing a structure that makes sense to those who use this text on a regular basis. By creating new sections and grouping chapters in a logical framework, this already-successful textbook has been strengthened.

This edition of the textbook is organized into six sections containing a total of 15 chapters. The sections are arranged by type of emergency for easier reference and a more reader-friendly approach to various emergencies that can occur in a dental practice. For example, Section Three: Respiratory Distress Emergencies contains chapters on respiratory emergencies that can happen in the dental setting. This organization will help the dental auxiliary student learn about related emergencies and the similarities and differences in how to handle them.

The new organization of this fourth edition is designed to ensure that those pursuing careers as dental professionals will have all the necessary skills and information to be prepared to effectively handle a medical emergency in the dental office with confidence.

Features

The fourth edition contains the following chapter elements:

Key Terms: Important terms are listed alphabetically at the beginning of each chapter and appear in the side margin with the definition upon the first appearance in the text.

Learning Outcomes: At the beginning of each chapter, these objectives address the concepts the reader should understand, and they allow immediate feedback on comprehension.

Test Your Knowledge: Short-answer questions are found throughout the chapters after core concepts have been introduced. These exercises are included to challenge the reader's knowledge and application of the material presented and to facilitate problem solving.

Emergency Basics: These boxed features, which facilitate understanding of important emergency protocols, warning signs and symptoms of an impending emergency, and more, are presented succinctly for quick and easy reference.

Summary: Each chapter includes a summary section that synthesizes chapter content covered and highlights main points.

Review Questions: Each chapter includes multiple choice and true/false questions to add another element of challenge for the reader, and to allow readers to double-check their progress and identify areas where further study is necessary.

Medical Emergency!: Engaging and thought-provoking case studies are located at the end of each chapter, after the review questions. These exercises inspire critical thinking and application of the material learned in the chapter to real-life emergency situations like those readers may face in the professional setting.

Glossary: The end of the textbook contains a complete listing of all key terms and their definitions for a quick and handy reference.

References: Found at the end of the textbook, this material provides students and instructors with resources that may be utilized for further inquiry.

New to the Fourth Edition

The fourth edition contains extensive content updates, including the most recent procedures for CPR, first aid, and treatment of airway obstruction. The process of updating the content and revamping the organization to a more user-friendly format has resulted in these changes in this edition:

- Six new section divisions have been added to organize the chapters by topic so that the material on medical emergencies pertaining to each topic can easily be found. The chapters appropriately fit into these sections for easy reference: Prevention, Altered Consciousness Emergencies, Respiratory Distress Emergencies, Cardiovascular Emergencies, Immune System Emergencies, and Legal Issues in Emergency Care.
- Chapter 2: Medical History has been added to address the importance of obtaining accurate medical history from patients in order to assess their likelihood of developing a medical emergency during a dental procedure.
- The Test Your Knowledge feature has been added to reinforce important concepts and to add another critical-thinking component to the chapters.
- In the Medical Emergency! sections, case studies have been expanded and updated to reflect possible situations that a dental auxiliary may face. Each case is tailored to the type of emergency that is the focus of the chapter.
- Key Terms, Learning Outcomes, and Review Questions all have been enhanced and updated with the chapter content changes to provide accurate and relevant study components.
- Many new figures and photographs provide visual illustrations of the content to help further comprehension of important procedures and equipment used during medical emergencies.
- References are now compiled comprehensively at the back of the textbook and have been updated to reflect the most recent industry standards and resources.

Also Available: Instructor Resources Online

(ISBN 978-1-1111-3861-5)

Spend less time planning and more time teaching with Delmar Cengage Learning's Instructor Resources to Accompany the *Emergency Guide for Dental Auxiliaries, fourth edition*. All Instructor Resources can be accessed by going to www.cengagebrain.com and creating a unique user log-in. The password-protected Instructor Resources include the following:

- An Instructor Manual, with answers to Test Your Knowledge questions and Review Questions, as well as additional materials for access at any time.
- A computerized test bank in ExamView® that makes and generates tests and quizzes in an instant. With a variety of question types, including short-answer and multiple choice questions, creating challenging exams will be no barrier in your classroom.
- Customizable instructor support slide presentations in PowerPoint® to direct classroom study on core chapter content.
- Additional case studies and exercises.

About the Author

Dr. Debra Jennings obtained her D.M.D. degree from the Medical University of South Carolina in Charleston during the class of 1990. During a 22-year experience at Trident Technical College, she taught in the Dental Hygiene and Expanded Duty Dental Assistant programs. During this time, she also taught a clinical course to first-year dental students at MUSC to enhance their knowledge of four-handed dentistry. Before attending the Medical University of South Carolina, Dr. Jennings earned dual degrees from the University of South Carolina in Anthropology/Criminal Justice and Biology/Chemistry. She has more than 35 years of practical experience in the dental field ranging from dental hygiene to dentistry. Dr. Jennings's many years of dental experience place her in the unique position of being at the pulse of modern teaching and dental practices. In addition to teaching, she has authored and edited various texts and articles for the dental community. When not in the academic arena, she volunteers with the Smiles for a Lifetime clinic that services low-income and immigrant populations. She is a South Carolina native and has lived in the Lowcountry for more than 30 years.

Dedication

To the memory of Mom and Dad, who supported me throughout my entire life.

Reviewers

Melanie Simmer-Beck, RDH, MS
Associate Professor & Senior Clinic Coordinator
University of Missouri—Kansas City School of Dentistry
Division of Dental Hygiene
Kansas City, Missouri

Teresa C. Bezak, BS, RDH, M.Ed.
Assistant Professor
School of Dental Medicine
University of Pittsburgh
Pittsburgh, Pennsylvania

Faith Y. Miller, RDH, MSED
Associate Professor
Dental Hygiene School of Allied Health
Southern Illinois University
Carbondale, Illinois

Joanne Pacheo, RDH, MAOB
Dental Hygiene Instructor
Fresno City College
Fresno, California

Lisa A. Scott, CDA, RDH, M.Ed.
Associate Professor
Allied Dental Education
Concord, New Hampshire

SECTION ONE

Prevention

This section deals with assessing the patient and the preparation of the office staff.

CHAPTER 1

Office Preparation

LEARNING OUTCOMES

Upon completion of this chapter, the student will be able to:

- Explain the role of the dental auxiliary during an office emergency
- Explain the importance of an office emergency routine
- Describe the functions of the auxiliary in relation to the emergency kit
- Identify the attachments used with an oxygen tank
- Explain the importance of the demand-valve resuscitator
- Demonstrate the operation of the oxygen tank

KEY TERMS

ampule

demand-valve
  resuscitator

emergency kit

flowmeter

nasal cannula

oxygen tank

regulator

Regardless of how much care is taken, not all dental office emergencies can be prevented. Therefore, should an emergency occur, the dental team must be prepared. In order to be prepared, the members of the dental team should have a well-planned and practiced emergency routine, have available all necessary equipment, and have appropriate emergency numbers posted at all phones. In addition, the entire staff should be trained in cardiopulmonary resuscitation (CPR) and up-to-date on the current CPR guidelines.

OFFICE EMERGENCY ROUTINE

To prevent a minor office emergency from becoming a serious or perhaps even a fatal event, it is important to have a thorough office emergency routine—a definitive plan that indicates the functions and responsibilities of each member of the dental team. Furthermore, it is essential that this routine be practiced so that when an emergency occurs, the established protocols can be carried out without hesitation.

Role of the Dental Auxiliary

Every dental office varies in how it designates responsibilities for each person; however, here are six responsibilities that may be delegated to the dental auxiliary:

1. *Notify the dentist of the emergency.* The dentist is responsible for everything in his or her office and must be notified immediately.
2. *Administer basic life support if necessary.* Basic life support consists of maintaining an open airway, providing rescue breathing, and providing external cardiac compressions. All auxiliaries should be able to provide basic life support if needed.
3. *Retrieve the emergency kit.* Once an emergency situation is identified, the emergency kit should be brought to the area immediately so that all the available equipment is ready for use.
4. *Retrieve the oxygen tank.* Oxygen is useful in most emergency situations. Have it available even if the cause or type of emergency has yet to be diagnosed.
5. *Retrieve hard backboard.* CPR cannot be performed effectively on a patient who is in a soft dental chair; therefore, many offices keep available a piece of board that fits in the back of the dental chair underneath the patient. This board should be brought to the patient's operatory and placed near the chair in case CPR becomes necessary. If a backboard is not available, the patient should be placed on the floor of the operatory before CPR is performed.
6. *Assist the dentist by preparing emergency drugs.* Although auxiliaries cannot legally administer drugs, in some states it is legal for them to prepare the drugs for the dentist to administer. Doing so, when allowed, is helpful in situations where several drugs must be given in succession.

Role of the Receptionist

The receptionist, although not usually in direct contact with the patient, has several responsibilities during an emergency:

1. *Have all emergency numbers updated and within easy reach.* It is an excellent idea to always keep these numbers posted close to the telephone.

2. *Notify the emergency medical service.* When contacting the emergency medical service, report the nature of the emergency and give explicit directions to the office. Here is a checklist for calling in an emergency:

   - State that your need for the rescue unit is an emergency and explain the nature of the emergency, if known.
   - Give the age of the injured person.
   - Specify the exact location.
   - Provide your name and telephone number.
   - Stay on the line until the operator instructs you to hang up.

3. *Go outside to direct emergency personnel into the office.* This saves valuable time once the rescue unit arrives.

4. *Keep patients in the waiting room calm.* If the emergency is serious, appointments for patients in the waiting room should be rescheduled. Depending on the circumstances, the receptionist can handle this while the patients are in the office or call them later. The waiting patients should be informed that there is an emergency situation but should not be given information concerning the patient's identity or the nature of the emergency.

These tasks do not have to be performed by the receptionist; anyone in the office may be assigned to do them. The important thing is that each person in the office has been informed about and understands exactly what his or her responsibilities involve during an emergency situation.

Practice Routine

Once each person in the office understands his or her responsibilities, the emergency routine must be practiced on a regular basis. An emergency situation should be simulated, with each person performing his or her assigned functions. A well-prepared staff handles an emergency much more efficiently than one that has not been prepared by performing practice drills.

TEST YOUR KNOWLEDGE

1. What is the role of the dental auxiliary during a dental office emergency?

2. What details should the dental receptionist or other person who calls for a rescue unit communicate to the emergency medical personnel?

EMERGENCY KIT

emergency kit
A kit containing the necessary medications and equipment required to treat an emergency.

There are several types of **emergency kits.** One type that is gaining in popularity is the homemade emergency kit. The homemade kit is usually assembled by the dentist with the help of physicians, pharmacists, and other medical personnel. This type of kit may be stored in a large tackle box, on a set of instrument trays, or in a cart specifically designed by a dental company for that purpose. The advantages of the homemade kit are:

1. The dentist knows exactly what is in the kit and is thus more likely to be able to use each piece of equipment and each drug proficiently.
2. The kit is designed by the dentist to meet his or her particular needs.

The second type of emergency kit is the manufactured kit. These kits, which are available from every major dental supply company, come in a variety of styles. The advantages of the manufactured kit are:

1. It comes in a carrying case that has compartments specially designed for each item.
2. It is designed specifically for dental office emergencies.
3. The kit is color coded to match the equipment or drugs with particular types of emergencies.
4. Some of these kits are available with prefilled syringes that allow for rapid emergency response.

TABLE 1-1   Sample Emergency Kit Contents
Ampule epinephrine or EpiPen®
Bronchodilator
Ammonia inhalants
Nitroglycerin tablets or spray
Bottle of atropine
Solu-Cortef® Mix-o-Vial
Sugar source (i.e., icing)
Automated external defibrillator (AED)
Ampule diazepam
Ampule Wyamine
Ampule Benadryl®
12-cc disposable syringe
3-cc disposable syringe
Tourniquet
12-gauge cricothyrotomy needle
Plastic airway

5. The kits often provide for automatic replacement of outdated medications.
6. These kits may come with emergency training videos.

The main disadvantage of the manufactured kit is that it can be an elaborate kit containing some equipment and drugs with which the dentist is not completely familiar.

The key to selecting the correct type of emergency kit for any dental office is to make sure it meets the dentist's needs. For example, in an office that is located a great distance from any medical facility, the dentist requires a fairly elaborate emergency kit, whereas a dentist whose office is located across the street from a hospital requires a minimal amount of emergency equipment.

See Table 1-1 for a list of the contents of a sample emergency kit and Figure 1-1 for a picture of possible contents.

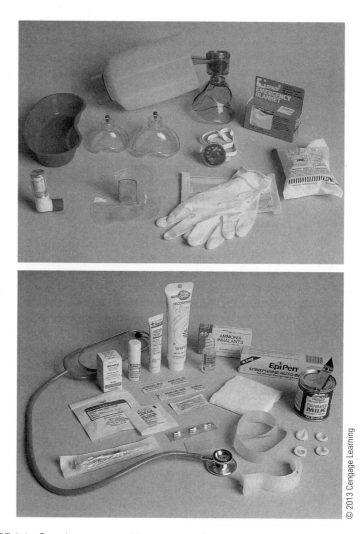

© 2013 Cengage Learning

FIGURE 1-1   Sample emergency kits commonly found in dental settings.

The Dental Auxiliary and the Emergency Kit

Auxiliaries may think that they do not need to be concerned about the emergency kit, since in most areas it is illegal for the auxiliary to use the majority of the items in the kit. In fact, auxiliaries should be thoroughly familiar with each piece of equipment and each drug in the emergency kit, since they can be of tremendous help during an emergency by promptly preparing, to the extent allowed, the correct drugs and equipment.

In addition, auxiliaries often are responsible for inspecting the emergency kit on a routine basis to check for broken equipment and expired or depleted drugs. This responsibility is assigned by the dentist as a part of the auxiliary's job description.

Drugs should always be kept updated. Administering an outdated drug during an emergency can prove fatal. If the dentist wishes, arrangements can be made with certain pharmaceutical companies to replace the drugs automatically before they reach their expiration dates. If such an arrangement is made, the dates should still be double-checked by the auxiliary to prevent any errors.

The auxiliary should become very familiar with the dental office's emergency kit. Kits ordered from manufacturers generally include instructions. However, if the kit was assembled by the dentist, the auxiliary may need to obtain special instructions from other sources. If the emergency kit contains controlled substances, a method of recording the administration of these drugs should be included in the kit.

ampule Sealed glass container that holds a single dose of medication.

Most manufactured kits contain drugs in single-dose **ampules** (Figure 1-2). These ampules are designed to make it easy for the dental team to prepare an injection during an emergency situation. To open the ampule, hold the ampule with both hands and break it open at the color-coded line. Be careful to hold the ampule upright when breaking it open to prevent spillage. Once the ampule is open, discard the top portion and load the syringe from the remaining portion of the ampule. Some emergency drugs, for example, the EpiPen®, come preloaded.

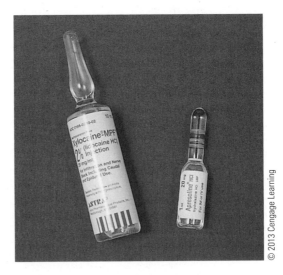

© 2013 Cengage Learning

FIGURE 1-2 Ampules.

The emergency kit should always be kept in one location that is known by everyone in the office, and it should be easily accessible to everyone in the office.

TEST YOUR KNOWLEDGE

1. What is an advantage of a homemade emergency kit?

2. Where should the emergency kit be located in a dental office?

OXYGEN TANK

oxygen tank
A cylinder that contains oxygen.

Oxygen is one item that can be easily administered by anyone trained in its use. It is extremely useful in most emergency situations except hyperventilation.

The oxygen comes in a cylinder. All **oxygen tanks** are green, which distinguishes oxygen from other gases. Cylinders range in size from very large to so small they can be carried in the hand (see Figure 1-3). Letters of the alphabet have been chosen to specify certain sizes of oxygen tanks; the best size for the dental office is the E cylinder. This cylinder contains about 650 liters of oxygen and provides 100 percent oxygen for 30 minutes of constant use.

Attachments

regulator
Attachment on an oxygen tank that allows oxygen to be released from the tank to the face mask or nasal cannula.

flowmeter
Attachment on the oxygen tank that controls the amount of oxygen that is delivered to the patient.

When the oxygen tank comes from the manufacturer, it consists only of the cylinder. A device known as a **regulator** must be attached to the tank so oxygen can be administered to the patient. The regulator is placed onto the tank to allow the pressure to be released at a reduced rate (Figure 1-4).

Once the regulator is in place, the flow of oxygen can be adjusted by using a **flowmeter** that controls the amount of oxygen given to the patient. Two main types of flowmeters are used. These are the bourbon gauge flowmeter and the pressure-compensated flowmeter. The bourbon gauge consists of a round dial that indicates the flow of oxygen in liters per minute. Although it is a pressure gauge and therefore may sometimes give inadequate readings when low amounts of oxygen are being administered, it is found on a majority of tanks used in dental offices and can be very functional. The pressure-compensated flowmeter consists of a vertical glass tube with a ball float that rises and falls with the flow of oxygen going through the tube. This gauge indicates the actual flow at all times. Because it depends on the force of gravity, it must always be operated in an upright position.

While the valves and gauges on the regulator and flowmeter are necessary to release oxygen from the tank, extra attachments also are required to administer oxygen to the

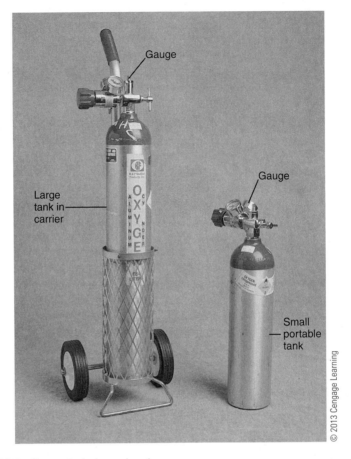

Gauge

Large
tank in
carrier

Gauge

Small
portable
tank

© 2013 Cengage Learning

FIGURE 1-3   Oxygen tanks in varying sizes.

nasal cannula
An attachment
that can be used
with the oxygen
tank; the cannula
fits into the
patient's nostrils
and delivers the
oxygen.

patient. A vast number of such attachments are available, ranging from **nasal cannulas** (see Figure 1-5) to full oxygen tents. A nasal cannula is used to deliver supplemental oxygen to a patient who needs respiratory help. However, a basic mask should be sufficient for administering oxygen during an emergency situation in a dental office.

Oxygen masks come in a variety of sizes designed for both adult and pediatric patients and should be available in every dental office. The mask must meet specific criteria to be effective. First, it must be the proper size and shape for the patient's face so as to provide a snug fit. Second, the mask should be made of a clear substance (Figure 1-6). It is imperative that the patient be monitored during oxygen administration to make sure he or she does not vomit into the mask and then aspirate the vomitus into the lungs; a clear mask makes this task easier. Furthermore, with a clear mask, the person administering the oxygen can tell when the patient has begun to breathe on his or her own because the mask will fog.

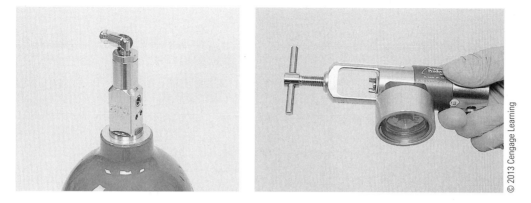

© 2013 Cengage Learning

FIGURE 1-4   The pins of the regulator must exactly match the holes in the tank's stem.

**demand-valve
resuscitator**
Attachment for
the oxygen tank
that can force
oxygen into
the lungs of a
nonbreathing
patient.

Another extremely important attachment for the office oxygen tank is the **demand-valve resuscitator.** The regular office oxygen tank is of no use on a patient who is not breathing, because there is no way to force the oxygen into the lungs. This is the function of the demand-valve resuscitator. The demand valve consists of a pushbutton, located on the face mask, that controls the flow of oxygen. When the button is pressed, oxygen goes through the mask with enough force to inflate the lungs, and is continually forced into the lungs until the valve reaches a preset pressure, at which point the oxygen stops. The demand valve is very beneficial during CPR because it provides 100 percent oxygen rather than the oxygen–carbon dioxide mix a human provides. Furthermore, once the patient starts breathing, the demand valve automatically provides oxygen when the person inhales and stops when the person exhales.

Other less-expensive items such as the Ambu bag may be used in place of the demand valve. The most important consideration is to have some mechanism available to force oxygen into the lungs of a nonbreathing patient.

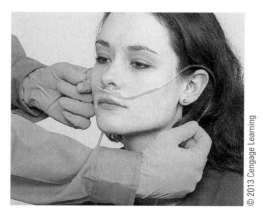

© 2013 Cengage Learning

FIGURE 1-5   Nasal cannula.

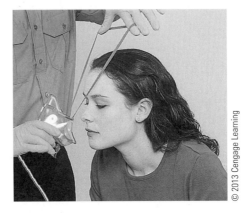

FIGURE 1-6   Clear face mask for oxygen administration; the mask should fit snugly to the patient's face for maximum effectiveness.

Operating the Tank

When operating an oxygen tank, follow these steps:

1. When opening a new tank, use the attached wrench to open the seal and release a little oxygen to clear dust and debris from the valves.
2. Attach the regulator and flowmeter, which are designed with specific grooves and holes that can attach only one way.
3. Open the regulator valve all the way and then turn it back one turn. This prevents someone from thinking it is closed and damaging the equipment by turning it the wrong way.
4. Adjust the flowmeter to the point at which it is releasing 4 to 6 liters of oxygen.
5. Check the face mask hose to make sure it is not twisted or knotted.
6. Place the mask over the patient's face. Make sure the mask fits the patient with a tight seal.
7. When oxygen therapy is completed, remove the face mask, turn the flowmeter to zero, and close the tank valve. Be sure to clean or dispose of the mask, depending on the manufacturer's instructions.

Precautions

Although oxygen is a relatively safe gas to administer, a few precautions should be followed in the dental office:

1. *Do not use oxygen near an open flame.* Oxygen is very flammable; although oxygen itself does not burn, it can cause a small flame to burn out of control.
2. *Eliminate grease and oil from the area, as any kind of grease or oil can cause oxygen to explode.* Make sure you do not have oil on your hands when you operate the tank. Do not store the tank near dirty, oily rags.

SUMMARY

Emergencies occur in even the best-prepared dental office. However, a staff that knows what its responsibilities are, has all the equipment available, and knows emergency procedures and how to use the emergency equipment often can prevent a minor emergency from becoming a major one.

REVIEW QUESTIONS

MULTIPLE CHOICE

1. During an office emergency, which of the following is not a function of the dental auxiliary?
   a. notify the doctor
   b. administer basic life support
   c. administer necessary drugs
   d. retrieve the emergency kit

2. All oxygen tanks are
   a. green.
   b. blue.
   c. red.
   d. yellow.

3. The amount of oxygen the patient receives is controlled by the
   a. regulator.
   b. demand valve.
   c. cylinder.
   d. flowmeter.

4. Grease or oil should not be used around oxygen because it will
   a. contaminate the oxygen.
   b. cause an explosion.
   c. block the valves.
   d. none of the above

5. Which of the following is/are true concerning the face mask on the oxygen tank?
   a. should be clear
   b. should form a tight seal
   c. should be made of metal
   d. both a and b

TRUE OR FALSE

_____   1. The emergency kit should be easily accessible to everyone in the office.

_____   2. Dental auxiliaries may administer oxygen if they are trained in its use.

_____   3. The expiration date on drugs found in the emergency kit can be checked only by
                  the dentist.

_____   4. An E-cylinder oxygen tank should be used in the dental office.

_____   5. When administering oxygen, the flowmeter should be set on 4–6 liters.

MEDICAL EMERGENCY!

CASE STUDY 1-1

A 45-year-old male presents with a medical history on which he states that he has heart problems. As dental treatment begins, the patient loses consciousness and goes into cardiac arrest. The doctor sends the auxiliary to the front to call for help while he goes to hook up the new oxygen cylinder that just arrived this morning. At the front desk, the assistant asks the receptionist to find the number for the emergency medical service. When the doctor and assistant return to the operatory, they begin two-person CPR with the patient in the dental chair.

Questions

1. List everything that was done incorrectly.

2. List the correct steps.

CASE STUDY 1-2

A 76-year-old female presents with a medical history on which she states that she has heart problems and diabetes. As the dental auxiliary begins to prepare the operatory, the patient loses consciousness. The dental auxiliary retrieves the emergency kit and administers several drugs to the patient. The dentist enters the operatory as the patient is regaining consciousness.

Questions

1. What did the dental auxiliary do incorrectly?

2. List the correct protocol.

CHAPTER 2

Medical History

LEARNING OUTCOMES

Upon completion of this chapter, the student will be able to:

* Name the basic components of a dental patient's medical history
* Name the basic components of a dental patient's dental history
* List the ASA classifications that are pertinent to the care of a dental patient
* Discuss the reasons for the importance of having a complete and accurate medical history for the dental patient
* Explain why confidentiality should be maintained on all information obtained from the dental patient
* Explain the importance of having an accurate, updated medical history for each dental patient
* Explain the technique for completing and updating the health history
* Explain the technique for utilizing the *Physician's Desk Reference (PDR)*
* List other sources for drug references that are available to the dental auxiliary

KEY TERMS

American Society of
   Anesthesiologists (ASA)
ASA Physical Status
   Classification System

assessment
Health Insurance Portability and
   Accountability Act (HIPAA)
medical history

*Physician's Desk Reference
   (PDR)*
protected health information
   (PHI)

Most dental office emergencies can be prevented through the use of information found on thorough medical histories. Dentists have found the easiest way to treat an emergency is to prevent it from occurring. This chapter discusses ways of gathering information from a **medical history** that may help prevent an emergency. In addition, the chapter will discuss the importance of maintaining confidentiality of information obtained from the patient.

medical history
Information obtained from a patient about past medical problems and medications that is useful in providing care to the patient.

There is a great variety of patient health history forms that are commercially available and can be purchased through various dental supply companies. Many dentists design their own forms to better suit the needs of their practice. Figure 2-1 provides an example of a medical history form.

MEDICAL HISTORY FORMAT

Regardless of what type of form the dental office uses, several components are essential. First, the form should include a section for general information, including such items as name, age, address, telephone number, and person to contact in case of an emergency. The patient's primary physician should also be listed in case medical consultations are required. Next, a detailed section should ascertain the past and present medical condition of the patient, especially conditions that can result in a potential emergency situation. This section should also include information on current prescribed medications, allergies, and past medical surgeries, and there should be a place for the patient to identify any conditions that he or she feels is important. Lastly, a dental history should be included to determine what dental treatment has been completed in the past and the results of that treatment.

The section on medical conditions is very important. Each condition should be listed by its common name so it will be easily understood by the patient. The format of the medical history form should be one that allows the patient to answer questions with a yes or no and has room for follow-up questions by the auxiliary. In addition, the format should be available in different languages to accommodate any non–English-speaking dental patients.

Completing the Medical History

The dental auxiliary or receptionist should always be available to help the patient complete the medical history. Some patients prefer to complete the forms by themselves; others may not understand some of the terminology and may require assistance. The dental auxiliary should verbally question the patient about any positive answers as well as any conflicting answers. Any medical conditions that the patient reports on the medical history should be reported to the treating dentist. Furthermore, the dental auxiliary should note any medical conditions that may result in a potential emergency event.

The dental auxiliary should maintain a professional and caring manner when questioning a dental patient about current and past medical circumstances.

MEDICAL HISTORY FORM

Please print.

Date: _____   Name_____

Mobile phone # _____   Email _____   Home phone # _____

Address _____

City_____   State_____   Zip Code _____

Occupation_____   Work Phone _____

Date of Birth_____   Height_____   Weight_____   Sex: M   F

Closest Relative_____   Phone # _____

If you are completing this form for another person, what is your relationship to that person?

_____

How did you find out about our clinic?_____

For the following questions, circle yes or no, whichever applies. Your answers are for our records only and will be considered confidential. Please note that during your initial visit you will be asked some questions about your responses to this questionnaire and there may be additional questions concerning your health.

1. Are you in good health?   Yes   No

2. Has there been any change in your general health within the past year?   Yes   No

3. What was the date of your last physical examination?   _____

4. Are you now under the care of a physician?   Yes   No

    If yes, what is the condition being treated?   _____

5. Your physician's name and address   _____

6. Have you had any serious illness, injury, or operation in the last five years?   Yes   No

    Have you been hospitalized in the last 5 years?   Yes   No

    If yes, what was the illness or problem?   _____

FIGURE 2-1   A sample medical history form with identification of important components such as personal information, past history of disease, and current prescriptions. (Continues)

7. Please place a check beside any of the following diseases or conditions you have now or have had in the past.

__ Damaged heart valves	__ Fainting spells	__ Respiratory problems
__ Artificial heart valves	__ Seizures	__ Arthritis
__ Heart murmur	__ Persistent diarrhea	__ Stomach ulcer
__ Rheumatic heart disease	__ Recent weight loss/gain	__ Kidney disease
__ Heart disease	__ Diabetes	__ Tuberculosis
__ Heart attack	__ Type I	__ Persistent cough
__ Angina	__ Type II	__ Low blood pressure
__ High blood pressure	__ Gestational	__ Sexually transmitted
__ Arteriosclerosis	__ Liver disease	disease
__ Stroke	__ Blood transfusion	__ Epilepsy
__ Chest pain upon exertion	__ Tumor or growth	__ Mental health disorders
__ Short of breath after mild	__ Bulimia	__ Cancer
exertion	__ Anorexia	__ Immune disorders
__ Swollen ankles	__ Hepatitis A, B, or C	__ Herpes (Cold sores/fever
__ Congenital heart defect	__ Jaundice	blisters)
__ Cardiac pacemaker	__ AIDS	__ Night sweats
__ Sinus trouble	__ HIV infection	__ Blood disorders
__ Hay fever	__ Thyroid problems	__ Sickle cell or other
__ Asthma	__ Emphysema	anemias
__ Use of a bronchodilator	__ Bronchitis	

8. Please place a check if you are allergic or have every had a reaction to:

__ Local anesthetics	__ Sulfa drugs	__ Codeine or other
__ Penicillin or other	__ Aspirin	painkillers
antibiotics	__ Iodine	__ Barbiturates, sedatives
__ Latex or rubber items		

9. Are you allergic to anything not listed? If so, what _____

10. Have you had any serious problem associated with any previous dental treatment?   Yes   No

11. Do you wear the following:

Contact lenses   Yes·   No

Removable dental appliances   Yes   No

12. Do you have any artificial implants, shunts, or artificial joint replacements?   Yes   No

If yes, does your physician recommend antibiotics before dental treatment?   Yes   No

13. Do you have any disease, condition, or problem not listed above that you think I should know about?   Yes   No

FIGURE 2-1   A sample medical history form with identification of important components such as personal information, past history of disease, and current prescriptions. (Continued)

14. Are you now taking or have you ever taken diet drugs prescribed by your doctor? (These would include, but are not limited to, Pondimin, Redux, Fen-phen, Phentermine, fenfluramine, dexfenfluramine.)   Yes   No

15. Are you taking Hormone Therapy?   Yes   No

16. Please provide the following information for any prescription and nonprescription medicine you are now taking:

Medicine's name	Beginning date	How often is the medicine taken?	Why do you take this medicine?

17. Circle if you are:

   Pregnant   Possibly pregnant, not sure   Nursing

18. Are you taking birth control pills or using other chemical means of birth control such as injections or implants (Implanon)?   Yes   No

19. What is your chief dental need or problem?   _____

I certify that I have read and understand all of the questions above. I acknowledge that my questions, if any, about the questions set forth above have been answered to my satisfaction. I will not hold the dentist, or any other member of his/her staff, responsible for any errors or omissions that I may have made in the completion of this form.

Patient's Signature _____**Date**_____

Parent/Guardian's Signature _____**Date**_____

© 2013 Cengage Learning

FIGURE 2-1   A sample medical history form with identification of important components such as personal information, past history of disease, and current prescriptions.

Health Insurance Portability and Accountability Act (HIPAA) Signed into law in 1996, a portion of this act establishes rules and regulations that define how information obtained from a patient can be circulated and to whom such information can be distributed with a patient's written consent.

protected health information (PHI) Under the Health Insurance Portability and Accountability Act (HIPAA), any information about health status, provision of health care, or payment for health care that can be linked to a specific individual.

assessment Review of the medical history and the likely side effects of any prescribed medications.

TEST YOUR KNOWLEDGE

1. What components should be present in the medical history?

2. How should a dental auxiliary help a non–English-speaking patient complete the medical history form?

Confidentiality of the Medical History

As with any other information obtained in the dental office, the information on the medical history is confidential. The information obtained on the medical history should be made available only to authorized users with the patient's full consent. In 1996, the **Health Insurance Portability and Accountability Act (HIPAA)** was signed into law. A portion of HIPAA establishes rules and regulations for the protection of **protected health information (PHI)**. The rules and regulations define how the information obtained from the patient can be circulated and to whom the information can be distributed with the patient's written consent.

Updating the Health History

Each time the patient returns to the office for a routine visit, the medical history should be updated. A person's medications and medical condition can change very rapidly, and it is extremely important to keep this information current.

TEST YOUR KNOWLEDGE

1. When should a medical history be updated?

2. What is PHI?

ASSESSMENT OF THE DENTAL PATIENT

In order to prevent an emergency from occurring, it is important for the dental auxiliary to take into account the dental patient's general health status. An **assessment** of the dental patient consists of reviewing the medical history and the likely side effects of any prescribed medications. After this information is evaluated, the patient can be placed into

American Society
of Anesthesiolo-
gists (ASA) An
association
of physicians,
primarily anesthe-
siologists, who
share a common
goal of improving
patient care
through education
and research.

**ASA Physical
Status Classifi-
cation System** A
six-category
physical status clas-
sification system
for assessing a
patient's risk before
treatment; usually
the dental team
deals with only the
first four categories.

TABLE 2-1	ASA Physical Status Classifications
ASA I	Normal healthy patient
ASA II	Patient with mild systemic disease
ASA III	Patient with severe systemic disease
ASA IV	Patient with severe systemic disease that is a constant threat to life
ASA V	Dying patient who is not expected to survive without an operation
ASA VI	Brain-dead patient whose organs are being removed for donor purposes

Source: American Society of Anesthesiologists, www.asahq.org/clinical/physicalstatus.htm.

a physical classification based on the **American Society of Anesthesiologists (ASA)** classification system shown in Table 2-1. When evaluating a patient's risk, the dental team is usually dealing with only the first four ASA classifications in the **ASA Physical Status Classification System.**

USING DRUG REFERENCE MANUALS

The dental auxiliary should research and record any information about the medications that are prescribed by the patient's physician or other health care provider. The dental auxiliary should note what medical condition each medication is prescribed for, and specifically call attention to any side effects of the medications, especially ones that have dental implications. Reviewing the medical history is extremely valuable to the entire dental team in understanding existing medical conditions, preventing improper mixtures of medications, and determining if there are restrictions on the type of treatment that may be provided to the patient.

All information determined by reviewing the patient's medical history should be described to the dentist so that he or she can ultimately determine how the patient's treatment will be accomplished to minimize the potential for emergencies. As a result of obtaining the information, it is sometimes necessary to consult the patient's physician or specialist to determine possible medical risks with any dental treatment.

Several sources may be utilized to obtain medication information. The dentist and staff should decide which source best meets the needs of their office.

*Physician's
Desk Reference
(PDR)* Published
book that
provides
information on
various drugs.

Using the *Physician's Desk Reference*

One drug reference source is the ***Physician's Desk Reference (PDR).*** The *PDR* is compiled annually and contains information provided by the drug manufacturers about a large variety of medications. Several sections are color coded and may be of value to the auxiliary. Complete instructions on how to use each section are provided at the beginning of the section.

The product identification section provides pictures of a wide variety of medications. Often patients come to the office with pill boxes containing a variety of medications, but they do not know the names of the medications or the conditions for which the medications have been prescribed. This section of the *PDR* allows the auxiliary to visually identify the medication.

The *PDR* is not the only general medication reference book. Another great resource to use for drug identification is the *Delmar Healthcare Drug Handbook,* which is updated annually as well.

Other drug reference sources are published for specific specialties in medicine as well as dentistry. These sources emphasize drug complications that are unique to the specialty referenced; for example, *Delmar's Mini Guide to Psychiatric Drugs* is focused on common prescriptions used in the field of mental health.

Finally, electronic versions of drug reference manuals are available through websites, CD/DVD sources, and applications. Caution should be used to determine the accuracy as well as the completeness of the information.

Even though it is ultimately the dentist's responsibility to make all decisions regarding the patient's medications, it is important for the auxiliary to know as much as possible about the patient to assist in providing proper treatment. The auxiliary should become familiar with the contents of the drug reference source selected and should utilize it regularly. It is extremely important to have an up-to-date resource, because medications change at such a rapid pace.

After the dental auxiliary has reviewed the medical history and the list of prescribed medications, a determination of whether the patient's medical history is positive or negative. A positive medical history would be one in which the patient presents with single or multiple medical conditions along with accompanying prescribed medications. A negative medical history would be one in which the patient presents with a no history of medical conditions and no prescribed medications.

TEST YOUR KNOWLEDGE

1. What ASA classifications would not usually be seen in a dental office setting?

2. What are examples of electronic drug reference sources?

SUMMARY

When a new patient enters the dental office, the staff and dentist seldom have any idea about the types of medical problems the patient has, so if an emergency were to arise, there would be no point of reference on which to base a probable diagnosis. The medical history informs the staff about possible problems for which to prepare as well as which drugs and treatments to avoid. When the dental team has all this information available, the doctor and staff have taken the first step toward preventing a serious dental office emergency.

REVIEW QUESTIONS

MULTIPLE CHOICE

1. If a dental patient has difficulty with English, the dental auxiliary should
   a. make an appointment for the patient when the services of an interpreter are available.
   b. have medical histories available in different languages.
   c. speak louder so that the patient will understand.
   d. suggest that the patient find a dentist who speaks his or her primary language.

2. Interviewing patients for their medical history requires
   a. special credentials.
   b. good communication skills.
   c. good computer skills.
   d. a lot of time and energy.

3. A normal healthy patient would be classified as
   a. ASA I.
   b. ASA II.
   c. ASA III.
   d. ASA IV.

4. A patient with a severe systemic disease would be classified as
   a. ASA I.
   b. ASA II.
   c. ASA III.
   d. ASA IV.

TRUE OR FALSE

_____ 1. The health history should be obtained only with emergency patients.

_____ 2. The health history should be updated each time the patient comes to the office.

_____ 3. The _Physician's Desk Reference_ should be replaced every year.

_____ 4. An ASA V classification patient would be commonly seen in a dental office for dental treatment.

MEDICAL EMERGENCY!

CASE STUDY 2-1

A 27-year-old female presents at the dental office for an initial exam. After the dental auxiliary reviews the medical history and records the vital signs, she notifies the dentist that the patient has a history of undercontrolled diabetes.

Questions

1. What ASA classification would fit this patient?

2. Would she have a positive or negative medical history? Why?

CASE STUDY 2-2

A 56-year-old male presents at the dental office for a restorative appointment. After reviewing the medical history and recording the vital signs, the dental auxiliary notifies the dentist that the patient has had a change in his medical history. He is no longer being treated for hypertension due to improvement through diet and exercise.

Questions

1.   What ASA classification would fit this patient?

2.   Would he have a positive or negative medical history? Why?

CHAPTER 3

Vital Signs

LEARNING OUTCOMES

Upon completion of this chapter, the student will be able to:

- Name the four primary vital signs
- Name two additional vital signs that may be necessary to monitor for patient treatment
- Demonstrate the technique for recording each of the four primary vital signs
- Explain the normal range of each of the four primary vital signs
- Explain why determining baseline vital signs is important in assessing a patient's health status

KEY TERMS

antecubital fossa	diastolic pressure	radial artery	stethoscope
baseline vital signs	hypertension	respiration rate	systolic pressure
blood pressure	pulse	sphygmomanometer	temperature
carotid artery			

baseline vital signs Vital signs (e.g., blood pressure, pulse, respiration rate, and temperature) that are recorded prior to treatment to help determine how the patient is responding during treatment.

Vital signs are clinical observations that are made to ascertain the patient's health condition, both physically and mentally. These clinical findings may provide the dental auxiliary and dentist with precise information on and clarification of how the patient may respond to treatment. Furthermore, the observation and recording of initial or **baseline vital signs** prior to any dental treatment can help the staff determine how the patient is responding during the dental procedure.

This chapter discusses ways of obtaining the four primary vital signs and the significance of these vital signs in the dental setting.

VITAL SIGNS

blood pressure The pressure the blood exerts on the walls of the arteries, the veins, and the chambers of the heart.

The human body has four vital signs that are important to measure: *blood pressure, pulse, respiration rate,* and *temperature.* Additionally, height and weight can be recorded especially if these observations are important in the patient's treatment. For example, in pediatric dentistry, height and weight for a child is necessary for the prescribing of medication.

BLOOD PRESSURE

hypertension Abnormally high pressure of the blood against the arterial walls.

systolic pressure Pressure on the arteries when the heart is beating, or working.

diastolic pressure Pressure on the arteries when the heart relaxes between beats.

stethoscope Instrument used to listen to the heart and chest sounds.

Blood pressure is the pressure the blood places on the walls of the arteries. When there is too much pressure on the arteries, the patient develops **hypertension,** also known as high blood pressure. Hypertension can result in serious conditions such as stroke or cardiac arrest. By measuring blood pressure, the dentist may recognize an undiagnosed condition of hypertension and can then refer the patient to a physician for a definitive diagnosis. The recognition of the hypertension status also can prevent an emergency from occurring in the dental office.

Two readings are recorded when blood pressure is measured. The first reading is the **systolic pressure,** a measurement of the pressure on the arteries when the heart is beating, or working. The second reading is the **diastolic pressure,** which is a measurement of the pressure on the arteries when the heart relaxes between beats. If a patient's blood pressure reading is 120/80, the 120 represents the systolic pressure, and the 80 is the diastolic pressure.

To measure blood pressure, two items are needed: a **stethoscope** and a **sphygmomanometer.** The sphygmomanometer, which consists of a gauge and an inflatable bag inside a cloth armband (see Figure 3-1), is available in a range of sizes designed to fit children and adults. The cuff should always be selected according to the patient's size rather than the patient's age.

sphygmomanometer
Instrument that consists of a gauge and an inflatable bag inside an armband; used to measure blood pressure.

TEST YOUR KNOWLEDGE

1. What four primary vital signs are recorded in a dental office?

2. What are two additional vital signs that may be recorded in the dental office?

A

Earpieces

Diaphragm

Bell

—Chest Piece

Rubber or Plastic Tubing

B

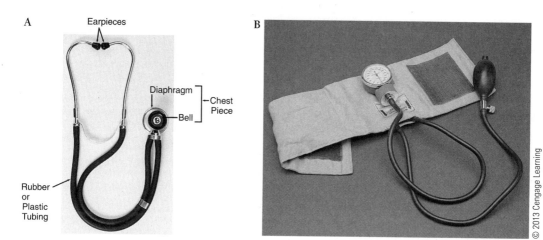

© 2013 Cengage Learning

FIGURE 3-1   (A) Stethoscope; (B) sphygmomanometer.

Technique

Blood pressure is measured by comparing the pressure in the artery with the air pressure in the armband using the following steps.

antecubital fossa Area approximately one inch from the elbow at which the stethoscope is placed in order to hear the pulse when measuring blood pressure.

Step 1
• Expose the patient's arm. An accurate blood pressure cannot be taken over any type of clothing.

Step 2
• Select the cuff size. Be sure to select a size that fits snugly around the patient's arm without being tight enough to stop the flow of blood. A cuff that is too large or too small may produce an inaccurate reading.
• Place the cuff approximately an inch above the **antecubital fossa** (Figure 3-2).

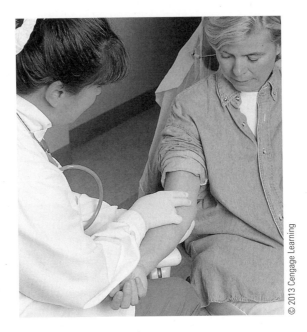

© 2013 Cengage Learning

FIGURE 3-2   Location of the antecubital fossa.

- Close the knob on the bulb by turning it clockwise. Make sure that the knob is not so tight as to prevent it from being easily turned with two fingers (Figure 3-3).

Step 3

radial artery An artery located in the forearm.

- Squeeze the bulb to pump air into the cuff until the pressure stops the flow of blood in the artery. This can be determined by palpating the **radial artery.** When no pulse is felt, the flow of blood has been stopped; make a note of this number. This is the palpatory radial systolic reading.
- Completely deflate the cuff.

Step 4

- Place the earpieces of the stethoscope into your ears. Make sure the earpieces are pointing toward the front of the head so that when they are placed in the ears, they follow the shape of the ear canal. This will enable you to hear the sound more efficiently.
- Reinflate the cuff so that the reading on the gauge is 20–30 mm Hg above the palpatory radial systolic reading.

Step 5

- Place the stethoscope over the brachial artery (Figure 3-4).
- Turn the knob on the bulb counterclockwise slowly to release the pressure in the cuff. If the pressure is released too rapidly, you will be unable to hear the pulse sound. If this occurs, release all the pressure in the cuff and begin the procedure again.
- As soon as the cuff is loose enough to allow the blood to pass through the artery, you should hear a pulse. At this point the reading on the gauge is the systolic pressure.

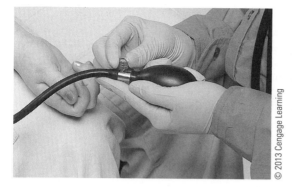

FIGURE 3-3 Close and open the knob on the blood pressure cuff.

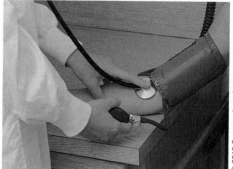

FIGURE 3-4 Placement of the stethoscope over the brachial artery.

Step 6

• Continue to release the pressure in the cuff until a pulse is no longer heard. At this point the blood is flowing freely, and the reading on the gauge is the diastolic pressure.

The technique described here is only one example of how to measure blood pressure. If you are in an office that utilizes a different technique, make sure you understand the steps involved and can perform the procedure accurately. Many dental offices use one of the different types of digital blood pressure cuffs that are available. When using a digital cuff, follow the manufacturer's instructions carefully to use the cuff effectively and to accurately record the reading.

TEST YOUR KNOWLEDGE

1. What is the first sound you hear when listening to blood pressure called?

2. What is the term for the second sound you hear when listening to blood pressure?

Normal Readings

Physicians once considered 120/80 the normal reading for an adult's blood pressure, but many now believe that a lower reading can be acceptable. To ensure an accurate reading and to determine what is normal for a particular patient, check the blood pressure over several visits. In addition, consult with the patient's physician if indicated. For example, if the dentist feels that the patient's health may be affected in any negative manner, a physician's consultation may be necessary.

When recording a patient's blood pressure, note the extremity utilized (e.g., arm or leg). Also note whether the right or left side has been used, as well as the position of the patient. Such a reading, for example, could be written as: 120/80 R. arm sitting.

See Table 3-1 for blood pressure categories used in the dental office setting.

TABLE 3-1	Blood Pressure Categories for Dental Offices			
	Systolic (mm Hg)		**Diastolic (mm Hg)**	
Normal	Less than 120	and	Less than 80	
Prehypertension	120–139	or	80–89	
Hypertension Stage 1	140–159	or	90–99	
Hypertension Stage 2	160 and above	or	100 and above	

Source: Adapted from the American Heart Association Guidelines, 2010.

RECORDING THE PULSE

pulse The regular expansion and contraction of an artery caused by the ejection of the blood from the left ventricle of the heart as it contracts.

carotid artery Artery located on either side of the neck; used to measure the pulse during an emergency.

The **pulse** is an important measurement to observe on each dental patient. Measuring the pulse gives the dentist a very good picture of what is taking place with the patient's cardiac rhythm. As with any vital sign, it is important to have a baseline reading for comparison in the event of an emergency.

The pulse can be measured at any major artery in the body. However, it is usually measured at either the carotid artery or the radial artery. The radial artery, located in the wrist area, is often the artery of choice for measuring the pulse during a routine examination (Figure 3-5). It provides both easy access and an accurate reading. The **carotid artery,** located on either side of the neck, should be used to measure the pulse during an emergency (Figure 3-6). When cardiac output is very low because of an emergency condition, the pulse may not be palpable at the radial artery (since the radial artery is peripheral, blood flow usually ceases in that area first). In this situation, measure the pulse at the carotid artery for more accuracy.

Technique

To record the pulse correctly, use the first and middle fingers in measuring it. Place the two fingers firmly over the artery. Placing the fingers too lightly will cause you to miss the beat of the pulse; pressing too tightly will cut off the blood supply, eliminating the pulse altogether.

Once the artery has been located, count each beat of the pulse for a full minute. Observing the second hand of a watch is mandatory. Although the rate or speed of the pulse is important, attention also must be paid to the rhythm (regular or irregular) and to the quality (bounding or thready). Each of these readings is very important to the dentist in diagnosing the problem during an emergency. Although normal pulse readings vary among patients, for an adult the average range is 60 to 80 beats per minute (bpm).

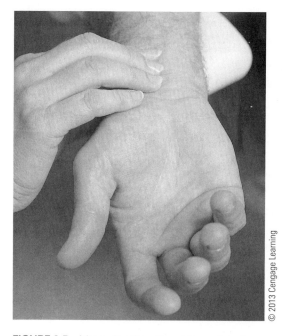

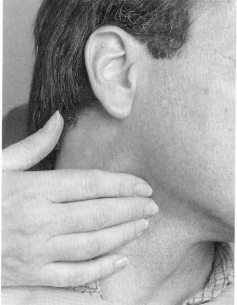

FIGURE 3-5   Measuring the pulse at the radial artery.   **FIGURE 3-6**   Measuring the pulse at the carotid artery.

RESPIRATION

respiration rate The number of times that a person inhales and exhales.

The measurement of respirations involves counting the number of times the patient breathes in and out in one minute. An unusual **respiration rate** is a signal of a possible emergency situation, such as hyperventilation or a cardiac problem.

To measure the patient's respirations accurately, make sure the patient is unaware that you are watching him or her breathe. By the patient being unaware of your actions, you can record a more accurate respiration rate. Continue holding the patient's wrist as though you are still measuring the pulse while you actually watch and count the rise and fall of the chest. As with the pulse, respirations should be measured for 60 seconds.

During cool weather when patients have on several layers of clothing, it is helpful to have the patient place one arm over the chest; the rise and fall of the arm then indicates the respirations. A normal range for respirations is 12 to 20 respirations per minute (rpm), although the rate can be dramatically different among certain groups of people, such as athletes.

TEMPERATURE

temperature The level of heat in the body.

A patient's body **temperature** is not usually measured in the dental office on a routine basis. However, if the dental team suspects that the patient may be ill, or if extensive surgery is to be performed, the dentist may request that the patient's body temperature be measured.

Use a thermometer to measure a patient's body temperature. An oral digital thermometer (Figure 3-7) is the type most often used in a dental office. However, a variety of thermometers and methods for measuring temperature are available, including digital or tympanic thermometers and temperature-sensitive strips. The dental staff should select an oral thermometer that best meets their needs.

Technique

The oral route is recommended for routine temperature measurement in the dental office. The technique described below is for use with an oral digital thermometer. If other methods are utilized, follow the manufacturer's instructions.

1. Remove the thermometer from the storage container and place the appropriate barrier over it to prevent contamination.

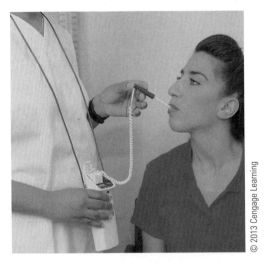

© 2013 Cengage Learning

FIGURE 3-7 A digital thermometer is the most commonly used type in dental settings.

2. Determine that the thermometer is activated.

3. Place the thermometer in the patient's mouth sublingually.

4. Instruct the patient to close the mouth and hold the thermometer in the mouth with the lips. Always caution the patient not to bite the thermometer.

5. Remove the thermometer from the patient's mouth and record the reading.

6. Clean the thermometer according to the manufacturer's instructions.

Normal Readings

The normal temperature reading for a child is 97–99 degrees; for an adult, 97–99 degrees; and for a geriatric patient (over 70 years old), 96–99 degrees.

SUMMARY

Vital signs such as blood pressure, pulse, respiration, and temperature are an excellent means of determining the patient's current medical status. In addition, the health history informs the dentist of past and present medical conditions. By obtaining all this information, the dentist and the auxiliary have taken the first step in assessing the patient's general health status.

REVIEW QUESTIONS

MULTIPLE CHOICE

1. Which of the following is/are considered a vital sign?
    a. temperature
    b. vision
    c. pulse
    d. both a and c

2. Which of these are needed to record blood pressure?
    a. sphygmomanometer
    b. thermometer
    c. stopwatch
    d. all the above

3. Which artery is used to measure blood pressure?
    a. femoral
    b. carotid
    c. radial
    d. brachial

4. Respirations should be measured for ___ seconds.
    a. 30
    b. 15
    c. 10
    d. none of the above

TRUE OR FALSE

_____   1. A normal range for respirations is 60 to 72.

_____   2. The thumb and first finger should be used to measure the pulse because they do not have a pulse of their own.

_____   3. Blood pressure may be recorded through any type of clothing.

MEDICAL EMERGENCY!

CASE STUDY 3-1

A 55-year-old female patient presents with a positive medical history. She indicates that she is taking prescribed medication for hypertension. After reviewing the medical history, the dental auxiliary obtains the patient's vital signs. The vital signs are: BP 120/70 L arm sitting, pulse 60 bpm, resp 18 rpm, and temp 98.6 degrees.

Questions

1.   For what medical condition is the patient taking prescribed medication?

2.   What additional information should be included with the blood pressure recording?

CASE STUDY 3-2

A 25-year-old male patient presents with a negative medical history. After reviewing the medical history, the dental auxiliary obtains the patient's vital signs. The vital signs are: BP 200/114 R arm sitting, pulse 90 bpm, resp 20 rpm, and temp 98.6 degrees.

Questions

1.   What should the dental auxiliary do after recording these vital signs?

2.   What medical condition could the patient have that he or she is not aware of?

SECTION TWO

Altered Consciousness Emergencies

This section deals with medical conditions that can result in the patient becoming disorientated, confused, or dizzy, thereby resulting in a medical emergency.

CHAPTER 4

Syncope

LEARNING OUTCOMES

Upon completion of this chapter, the student will be able to:

- Define syncope
- Describe the causes of syncope
- Describe the physiology of syncope
- Explain ways to prevent syncope
- List the signs and symptoms of syncope
- Demonstrate the treatment for syncope

KEY TERMS

nonpsychogenic	psychogenic	syncope
presyncope	supine position	Trendelenburg position

syncope
Fainting.

The most common life-threatening emergency that may be experienced in the dental office is **syncope** (better known as the common faint), a loss of consciousness caused by a decrease in the blood flow to the brain. Although syncope is a fairly common occurrence, if not promptly corrected it can lead to death. As a result, it has been suggested that all episodes of unconsciousness should be treated as a life-threatening emergency until otherwise diagnosed.

CAUSES

psychogenic
Psychological causes of a condition.

nonpsychogenic
Physical, nonpsychological causes of a condition.

Syncope is most often caused by some form of stress—physical, emotional, or both. For descriptive purposes, these causes have been categorized as either *psychogenic* or *nonpsychogenic*. **Psychogenic** factors are psychological causes; **nonpsychogenic** factors are physical causes.

Psychogenic factors include fear, pain, emotional upset, and anxiety that can be specifically related to the dental office in the following ways:

1. Most dental patients have some degree of fear about dental treatment. When this fear becomes overwhelming and unmanageable, it can become a psychogenic cause of syncope.
2. All the modern advances have come close to making routine dentistry a painless experience. Even so, in some situations (e.g., inadequate anesthesia), pain may be experienced. This type of sudden pain may cause syncope.
3. Unfortunately, dentists often have to inform patients of a poor prognosis. Bad news can sometimes trigger an emotional upset in a patient severe enough to cause syncope.

Psychogenic factors are the most common causes of syncope in the dental office.

Nonpsychogenic factors include hunger, poor health, and remaining in an upright position for a long period. Although nonpsychogenic factors can certainly cause syncope, they are experienced in the dental office much less often than psychogenic factors.

PHYSICAL CHANGES RESULTING IN SYNCOPE

Once certain psychogenic or nonpsychogenic factors are present, changes within the body may result in syncope. First, the body experiences some type of stress (e.g., pain or fear). As a result, certain products in the body trigger a reaction that causes a dilation of the vascular bed, resulting in a large amount of blood being pumped—mainly to the muscles of the arms and legs (the "fight-or-flight" syndrome). Since the patient remains stationary in the dental chair, this extra blood is not recirculated adequately and tends to pool in the arms and legs, resulting in a deficiency of blood to the heart, and thus a lack of oxygenated blood being supplied to the brain. As a result of the brain's deprivation of adequate oxygen, a state of unconsciousness occurs.

SIGNS AND SYMPTOMS

Syncope usually occurs with the patient in an upright position, such as sitting upright in the dental chair. Syncope is a relatively slow-occurring problem, usually passing through two different stages, in each of which the patient exhibits distinctive signs and symptoms.

presyncope
First stage of syncope; stage prior to the actual loss of consciousness.

Presyncope, the first stage, precedes actual loss of consciousness. During this stage the patient is pale and covered in cold sweat, and may complain of feeling hot, dizzy, or nauseated. Vital signs at this time show a slight decrease in blood pressure and a very rapid increase in pulse. The decrease in blood pressure is due to the dilation of the vessels, and the increase in pulse rate is due to the heart working so hard to send the extra blood to the brain. The heart can work this hard only for a short period of time. Once it tires, it no longer circulates a sufficient amount of blood. Therefore, the blood pressure and pulse rate drop rapidly immediately before the patient advances to the syncope stage.

Syncope, the next stage, consists of the actual loss of consciousness. During this stage, the patient exhibits a death-like appearance, the breathing may be shallow and gasping, slight convulsive movements may be present, pupils are dilated, and loss of bladder control may occur. Vital signs monitored at this time show a very low blood pressure and a slow, thready pulse.

See Emergency Basics 4-1 for a summary of the signs and symptoms of presyncope and syncope.

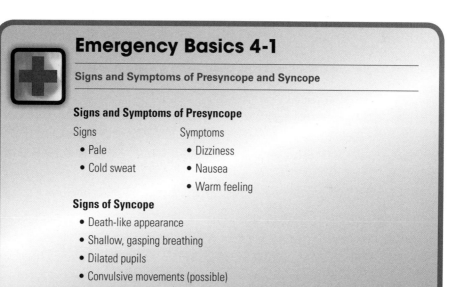

Emergency Basics 4-1

Signs and Symptoms of Presyncope and Syncope

Signs and Symptoms of Presyncope

Signs
- Pale
- Cold sweat

Symptoms
- Dizziness
- Nausea
- Warm feeling

Signs of Syncope
- Death-like appearance
- Shallow, gasping breathing
- Dilated pupils
- Convulsive movements (possible)
- Possible loss of bladder control

TEST YOUR KNOWLEDGE

1. What is an initial sign that could indicate the dental patient is experiencing syncope?

2. What is the primary cause of syncope in dental patients?

TREATMENT

Trendelenburg position
Position in which the patient is supine with the feet higher than the head.

supine position
Lying horizontally on the back.

First, remain calm. During syncope, as in all emergencies, the dental team must remain calm and in control. The patient who experiences syncope and revives to see a very nervous and upset support group could very easily have a relapse.

As soon as you suspect that a patient is experiencing syncope, stop all dental treatment. The traditional notion of having the patient place his or her head between the knees is no longer accepted as a means of treatment. Placing the head between the knees makes it more difficult to breathe; in this position, the patient's brain does not receive adequate oxygen—which is what caused the episode in the first place. Instead, place the patient in the **Trendelenburg position** (Figure 4-1). The Trendelenburg position is a **supine position** with the feet slightly elevated. Since most dental patients are already in the supine position, this position is easily achieved by slightly lowering the back of the chair. Placing the patient in this reclining position helps alleviate syncope because gravity is no longer a factor in getting blood to the brain.

If the patient loses consciousness in the waiting room or hallway, place the patient supine on the floor and elevate the legs slightly. This may be accomplished by placing an object such as a chair, coat, pillow, or a similar elevating device under the feet or simply by holding the legs in an elevated position.

Properly positioning the patient is the most important step in treating syncope and should be followed in every case except when dealing with a pregnant patient. If a

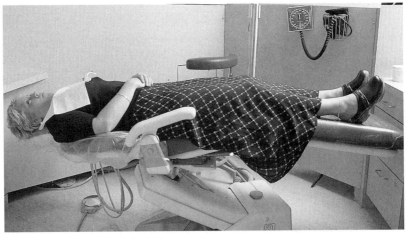

© 2013 Cengage Learning

FIGURE 4-1 The Trendelenburg position is the most effective position in which to place a patient experiencing syncope because it uses the force of gravity to allow blood to flow to the brain.

pregnant patient is placed in the Trendelenburg position, the weight of the fetus pressing against the diaphragm may inhibit breathing. Therefore, pregnant patients should be placed on their side before elevating the feet.

Once properly positioned, the patient should recovery rapidly. If recovery does not occur right away, the next step is to make sure the patient has an open airway. When a person loses consciousness, the muscles of the tongue relax and the tongue may fall to the back of the throat, blocking the airway. When the airway is blocked, no oxygen goes to the brain, and the patient could die. To open the airway, utilize the head tilt/chin lift techniques.

After the airway is opened, the patient should begin to breathe on his or her own. If this does not happen, other causes of unconsciousness must be considered, and more extensive treatment may be required. An ammonia capsule may be cracked and passed quickly back and forth under the patient's nose for one to two seconds to help stimulate breathing. However, the ammonia capsule should not be left in place for an extended period of time, as it can irritate the nasal membranes and cause difficulty in breathing. Pure oxygen via a full face mask also may be administered to aid in breathing and recovery. The vital signs should begin to return to their baseline readings during recovery.

Anything that can be done to help make the patient more comfortable during and following a syncope episode should be done. This includes loosening tight clothing, placing a cold towel on the forehead, or providing some type of covering if the patient complains of being cold once he or she begins to recover.

Recovery from a Syncopial Episode

On first recovering from an episode of syncope, a patient may be slightly confused and upset. The situation should be explained to the patient in a calm, reassuring manner. Some patients may be embarrassed by the episode; if so, extra efforts should be made to put the patient at ease.

A patient who has experienced a syncopial episode may faint again soon after recovery. Therefore, it is very important to remove any predisposing stimuli such as needles, blood, and the like from the patient's sight. The doctor and patient will have to decide whether dental treatment will continue, but whatever the decision, the patient will need some time to recover and should be kept calm and quiet. Also, the patient should not be left unattended. A patient who has lost consciousness in the dental chair should not be moved until fully recovered. If the episode has occurred in the waiting room or hallway, it is best, once consciousness has returned, to move the patient to a more appropriate area in which to recover.

Once the patient has recovered completely, all the information concerning the episode should be documented in the patient's chart, including the signs and symptoms exhibited and the treatment provided. An example of treatment for syncope is shown in Emergency Basics 4-2.

Emergency Basics 4-2

Treatment for Syncope

1. Remain calm
2. Place patient in Trendelenburg position (or if patient is pregnant, on her side)
3. Maintain open airway
4. Use ammonia capsule
5. Furnish oxygen
6. Monitor vital signs
7. Make patient comfortable
8. Record all information in patient chart

TEST YOUR KNOWLEDGE

1. What is the most important step in the treatment of a patient experiencing syncope?

2. What is different about the treatment of a pregnant patient who experiences syncope?

PREVENTION

If the signs and symptoms of presyncope are noted early enough, in most instances, you can prevent the patient from ever advancing to the full syncope stage. When such signs and symptoms as cold sweat, nausea, or dizziness are present, stop dental treatment and place the patient in the Trendelenburg position. Also try to remove or alleviate whatever caused the patient distress in the first place. In most cases, patients will recover completely.

Furthermore, it is possible to prevent any signs and symptoms of any phase of syncope. Since fear and anxiety are the most common causes of syncope in the dental office, the easiest way to prevent syncope is to alleviate such fear and anxiety. This can be achieved by doing everything possible to make the patient comfortable, which may include talking with the patient, providing a bright, cheery atmosphere, and alleviating unpleasant sounds and smells associated with the dental office. In some cases it might be helpful to premedicate a patient to alleviate extreme anxiety.

Syncope also may be prevented by maintaining a thorough, updated health history on each patient. The patient who has a history of syncope is highly likely to experience it during a dental visit. If the staff can find out what causes that person to faint, extra precautions can be taken to prevent the patient from experiencing these conditions.

SUMMARY

By being familiar with the patient's history and taking extra effort to reduce stress in the dental office, the auxiliary can prevent most cases of syncope from ever occurring. However, in the event syncope does occur, the well-trained auxiliary can correct a potentially life-threatening emergency by following the basic treatment procedure of placing the patient in the correct position, maintaining an open airway, and administering ammonia and oxygen.

REVIEW QUESTIONS

MULTIPLE CHOICE

1. The main cause of syncope is
    a. hunger.
    b. stress.
    c. excitement.
    d. overactivity.

2. Which of the following conditions would be considered a psychogenic factor of syncope?
    (1) hunger
    (2) fear
    (3) pain
    (4) poor health
      a. 1, 2, 3
      b. 1, 2
      c. 2, 3
      d. 3, 4

3. During which stage of syncope would the patient complain of being dizzy and hot?
    a. syncope
    b. presyncope
    c. a and b
    d. none of the above

4. Which of the following are sign(s) of the syncope stage?
    (1) cold sweat
    (2) nausea
    (3) dilated pupils
    (4) dizziness
      a. 2, 4
      b. 1, 3
      c. 3
      d. 1

5. Placing a patient in the supine position with the feet elevated is known as the _____ position.
   a. Trendelenburg
   b. prone
   c. recovery
   d. syncope

6. The purpose of the ammonia capsule is to
   a. burn the nasal passages.
   b. stimulate breathing.
   c. provide 100 percent oxygen.
   d. none of the above

TRUE OR FALSE

_____ 1. Syncope is a life-threatening emergency.

_____ 2. Once a patient has experienced syncope, he or she is a likely candidate for it to recur.

_____ 3. Nonpsychogenic factors are the most common cause of syncope in the dental office.

_____ 4. Syncope is a loss of consciousness due to an increase in the flow of blood to the brain.

_____ 5. Fear is an example of a psychogenic factor causing syncope.

_____ 6. During presyncope there is a decrease in blood pressure and an increase in pulse rate.

_____ 7. A good treatment for syncope is to have the patient place the head between the knees.

_____ 8. Since the patient is unconscious, it is not important for the dental team to remain calm while treating syncope.

_____ 9. If presyncope is recognized and treated properly, most instances of syncope can be prevented.

_____ 10. The patient may leave the office immediately after recovering from syncope.

MEDICAL EMERGENCY!

CASE STUDY 4-1

A 32-year-old female presents with a positive medical history. She is six months' pregnant and has come to the dental office because she has had some pain in the maxillary right central. While waiting for the dentist to come into the operatory, she complains of feeling hot and a little dizzy. A few minutes later she loses consciousness. The auxiliary assumes the patient is suffering from syncope. She places the patient in the Trendelenburg position, administers oxygen, and passes an ammonia capsule underneath the patient's nose.

Questions

1. What should the auxiliary have done when the patient first began to complain of feeling hot and dizzy?

2. Why should the patient not have been placed in the Trendelenburg position?

3. What position should this patient have been placed in?

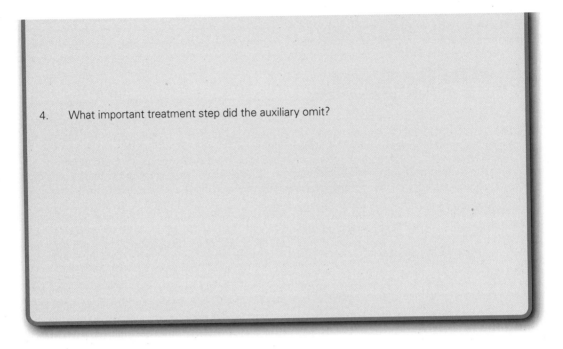

4.   What important treatment step did the auxiliary omit?

CASE STUDY 4-2

A 45-year-old male presents with pain in the maxillary right molar. He is in good general health, but has not seen a dentist for 10 years. While waiting in the treatment room, the dental auxiliary notices that the patient has begun to sweat profusely. As the auxiliary questions the patient, he tells her that he feels dizzy and nauseous.

Questions

1.   What condition is the patient most likely experiencing?

2.   What treatment should be done for this patient?

3.   What could have been done to prevent this experience?

CHAPTER 5

Seizure Disorders

LEARNING OUTCOMES

Upon completion of this chapter, the student will be able to:

- Define epilepsy
- Explain some of the causes of epilepsy
- Describe what takes place during a tonic-clonic (grand mal) seizure
- Define an absence (petit mal) seizure
- Define a partial (focal or localized) seizure
- Describe status epilepticus
- Explain the treatment of an epileptic seizure
- Describe some possible dental implications of epilepsy
- Explain how some epileptic seizures may be prevented

KEY TERMS

absence (petit mal)
  seizure
aura
clonic

Dilantin gingival
  hyperplasia
epilepsy
Jacksonian seizure

partial (focal or
  localized) seizure
status epilepticus
tonic

tonic-clonic (grand mal)
  seizure

epilepsy A type of seizure disorder that affects people for a variety of reasons and is not selective as to ethnicity, age, or gender.

A seizure occurs as a result of a sudden discharge of electrical energy somewhere in the central nervous system caused by an imbalance among the neurons of the brain. The area of the brain that is affected determines the type of seizure the patient experiences. **Epilepsy** is a type of seizure disorder that affects people for a variety of reasons and is not selective as to ethnicity, age, or gender.

CAUSES

In the majority of cases the cause of epilepsy is unknown, but in a few types of epilepsy the cause of the disease has been determined. First, an accident, such as a fall or a car accident, that traumatizes and damages the brain can result in the person developing a seizure disorder or epilepsy. Epilepsy also may be caused by injury during birth, a severe infection, or a fever high enough to cause damage to the brain. Furthermore, heredity plays a role in the cause of epilepsy. It has been documented that if both parents have epilepsy, the chances of their children or descendants developing a seizure disorder are greatly increased.

TYPES OF SEIZURES

tonic-clonic (grand mal) seizure An epileptic seizure characterized by generalized involuntary muscular contraction and cessation of respiration followed by tonic and clonic spasms of the muscles.

aura A sight, sound, or smell unique to an individual before experiencing an epileptic seizure.

tonic Movements characterized by continuous tension or contraction of muscles that are associated with a tonic-clonic (grand mal) seizure.

Epileptic seizures are usually identified by the actions that occur while the seizure is in progress. This section will discuss the different types of seizures that can occur. Types of seizures covered are:
- Tonic-clonic (grand mal) seizure
- Absence (petit mal) seizure
- Partial (focal, localized) or Jacksonian seizure

Tonic-Clonic (Grand Mal) Seizure

Tonic-clonic (grand mal) seizures are the most common. The term *tonic-clonic* is often used in place of *grand mal* in reference to the body movements the patient makes during the seizure. The tonic-clonic seizure can be divided into three phases: prodromal, convulsive, and postictal (see Emergency Basics 5-1).

Prodomal Phase The first phase is the prodromal phase, which includes the period before the actual seizure occurs. During this period, the patient may experience slight personality changes. These are usually so subtle that they are noticed only by people who are very close to the patient, such as family members. Some patients may experience an **aura** during this phase. The aura may consist of a certain smell, a flash of light, or a certain noise. Auras are usually unique to the individual and occur just before the patient advances to the convulsive phase.

Convulsive Phase The convulsive phase consists of the actual **tonic** and **clonic** movements. The patient loses consciousness, falls down, and in some instances gives out the epileptic cry. This cry results from the air rushing out of the lungs as the patient loses consciousness. Next, the patient's body stiffens and becomes rigid—the tonic stage. As the

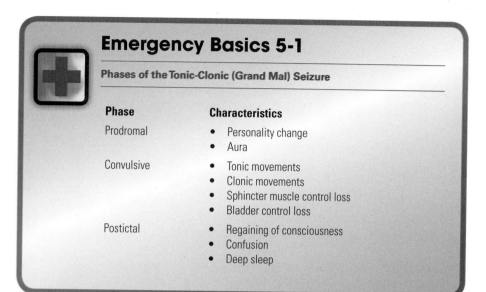

Emergency Basics 5-1

Phases of the Tonic-Clonic (Grand Mal) Seizure

Phase	Characteristics
Prodromal	• Personality change • Aura
Convulsive	• Tonic movements • Clonic movements • Sphincter muscle control loss • Bladder control loss
Postictal	• Regaining of consciousness • Confusion • Deep sleep

clonic Movements marked by contraction and relaxation of muscles that are associated with a tonic-clonic (grand mal) seizure.

patient passes into the clonic stage, the body begins to jerk violently. There may be foaming at the mouth, caused by air mixing with blood and saliva. The patient also may not be able to control bladder or sphincter muscles.

Postictal Phase The final phase of the grand mal seizure consists of the postictal phase. During this phase, the actual seizure is over, and the patient should slowly begin to regain consciousness. The patient may be confused about what happened and about where he or she is. In addition, the patient may need to sleep for a while in order to recover.

Absence (Petit Mal) Seizure

absence (petit mal) seizure An epileptic seizure characterized by a sudden momentary loss of consciousness occasionally accompanied by minor twitching.

The second type of seizure is the **absence (petit mal) seizure.** The term *absence seizure* is used because it best describes what occurs during the seizure. The patient experiencing an absence seizure loses awareness of their surroundings for a very short time. He or she may have a blank stare, twitch, or blink rapidly. This type of seizure, which may come and go without anyone around the patient realizing that he or she is experiencing a seizure, is most often seen in children and is often misdiagnosed as a behavioral problem in school-age children.

Partial (Focal or Localized) Seizure

partial (focal or localized) seizure Convulsive movements associated with epilepsy occurring on one side of the body only.

The third type of seizure is the **partial (focal or localized) seizure.** A simple partial seizure is sometimes classified as a **Jacksonian seizure.** This type of seizure involves only one hemisphere of the brain, so the patient may experience a jerking movement of only one part of the body, such as a leg or arm, rather than convulsive movements of the entire body. In addition, a person having this type of seizure may appear to be in a trance-like state and may fidget, pick at clothing, wander around, or exhibit continuous lip smacking. In some cases, a partial seizure may progress into a full tonic-clonic seizure.

Figure 5-1 shows the differences between a partial and a tonic-clonic seizure.

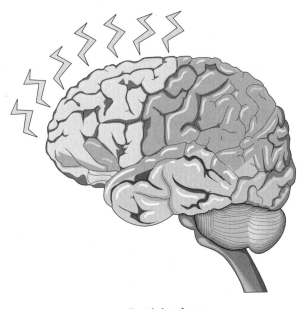

Partial seizure

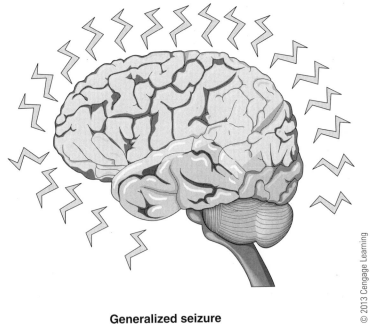

Generalized seizure

FIGURE 5-1   As shown, a partial seizure affects only a portion of the brain versus a tonic-clonic seizure that is characterized by chaotic firing all over the brain.

Jacksonian seizure A simple partial (focal or localized) seizure.

status epilepticus Situation in which a person experiences one seizure after another or one continuous seizure.

TEST YOUR KNOWLEDGE

1. What is the most common type of seizures seen in the dental office?

2. In what phase would a patient experience an aura?

3. Why do patients experiencing a seizure produce an "epileptic cry"?

Status Epliepticus

The most dangerous type of seizure is **status epilepticus,** which is extremely dangerous as it causes death in 10 percent of all cases. During status epilepticus, the patient experiences either one continuous seizure or one seizure after another. The body cannot handle this condition, and therefore the patient is in a life-threatening situation.

See Emergency Basics 5-2 for a summary of the different types of seizures and their characteristics.

Emergency Basics 5-2

Types of Seizures

Tonic-clonic (grand mal) seizure
- Aura
- Tonic/clonic movements
- Unconsciousness

Absence (petit mal) seizure
- Blank stare
- Twitching
- Rapid blinking
- Short duration

Partial (focal or localized) seizure
- Jerking movements of one body part
- Trance-like state
- Fidgeting

Status Epilepticus
- Continuous seizure
- Life-threatening

TEST YOUR KNOWLEDGE

1. What condition is a patient experiencing when several epileptic seizures occur one after the other?

2. What are some known causes of seizures?

3. What type of seizure may result in the patient having tonic and clonic movements?

TREATMENT

Witnessing an epileptic seizure can be traumatic. When treating a patient experiencing a seizure, try to stay calm and remember that the seizure is usually brief and not life-threatening, and that the patient requires very little care.

As far as the dental team is concerned, the main method of treatment for a seizure is to keep the patient from injuring himself or herself during the actual seizure and to provide supportive help once the seizure is over. Follow these steps:

1. Remove all dental objects from the patient's mouth.
2. Remove all dental equipment on which the patient may injure himself or herself, but if possible do not move the patient. If a patient is in the dental chair and certain objects on which the patient could be injured cannot be moved, move the patient to the floor.
3. Remove glasses and loosen tight clothing such as neckties. Dentures or partial dentures should remain in the patient's mouth unless they are causing an airway obstruction.
4. Call emergency medical services (EMS). There is always a possibility of injury during a seizure. Furthermore, EMS needs to be on-site in case the patient stops breathing and does not recuperate immediately or the seizure seems to pass from one episode right into the next.
5. Do not force anything into the patient's mouth. Placing an item into the patient's mouth may cause injuries to the oral cavity, such as lacerations or broken teeth. In addition, dental personnel may get bitten.
6. Do not restrain the patient. If you try to restrict the patient from making the convulsive movements, which are forceful, you can injure the patient's muscles or tendons, or you may be hit by a flailing arm or leg. The patient needs to be restricted only to the point of preventing injury, for example, to prevent the patient from hitting his or her head on the floor or injuring extremities on a nearby object. A pillow or soft towel should be placed under the patient's head or around an exposed extremity to prevent injury.

7. Once the seizure has ended, turn the patient on one side so that any secretions will not be aspirated. Remember that, above all else, an open airway must be maintained during the entire seizure.

8. The patient who begins to regain consciousness needs reassurance and may be confused about what happened, what day it is, and where he or she is. Also, most patients will be embarrassed by the episode; you should do whatever possible to alleviate this embarrassment and to help the patient maintain dignity.

9. Do not give the patient anything to eat or drink until he or she is fully alert.

10. The patient should be given plenty of time to rest and recover. Some patients go into a deep sleep for several hours. The patient should be placed in an appropriate area and allowed to remain there until fully recovered.

Emergency Basics 5-3 summarizes these steps for the treatment of a patient having a seizure.

TEST YOUR KNOWLEDGE

1. What treatment would not be indicated for a patient experiencing a seizure?

2. How can the dental auxiliary determine if the patient is beginning the prodromal stage?

3. How can the dental health care provider protect the patient's head during a tonic-clonic seizure?

Emergency Basics 5-3

Treatment of a Seizure

1. Remove dental materials from the patient's mouth.
2. Remove objects that may injure the patient.
3. Remove glasses and loosen clothing.
4. Call EMS.
5. Do not restrain the patient.
6. Place the patient on one side once the seizure is over.
7. Reassure the patient.
8. Do not give the patient anything to eat or drink.
9. Let the patient recover.

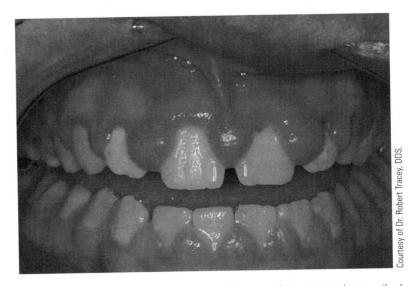

Courtesy of Dr. Robert Tracey, DDS.

FIGURE 5-2   Dilantin gingival hyperplasia is a side effect of the commonly prescribed seizure disorder drug Dilantin.

DENTAL IMPLICATIONS OF SEIZURE DISORDERS

The dental office is a likely setting for the occurrence of an epileptic seizure, just as it is for many other stress-related emergencies. Furthermore, the dental office may have to deal with special situations related to epilepsy or other seizure disorders.

Dilantin®, one of the drugs commonly given to treat seizure disorders, may produce a condition known as **Dilantin gingival hyperplasia,** in which the gingival tissue grows at a rapid rate and in some cases covers the teeth completely. In such extreme cases, the tissue is surgically removed. Figure 5-2 demonstrates the effect of Dilantin on a patient's gingival tissue.

Dilantin gingival hyperplasia
Overgrowth of gingival tissue that results from the intake of Dilantin.

TEST YOUR KNOWLEDGE

1. What anticonvulsant medication has dental implications?

2. What must be done in extreme cases to correct gingival hyperplasia caused by this anticonvulsant medication?

PREVENTION

Most of the causes of seizures are still unknown, and in these circumstances it is impossible to prevent people from developing seizure disorders. However, in the majority of cases, seizure disorders can be controlled and seizures prevented through the administration of an anticonvulsant, such as the commonly used Dilantin, discussed earlier. An anticonvulsant medication cannot cure a seizure disorder, but it can control the seizures in about 75 percent of patients.

If a seizure takes place in the dental office, try to remember what happened before the attack occurred, as this may help you determine what triggered the seizure episode. For example, was a material being used that had a distinct odor, or did an instrument emit a particular sound? By making this determination, it may be possible to prevent some seizures from occurring in the dental office in the future.

Seizures can be triggered in some patients by extremely stressful situations. To many people the dental office provides just this type of situation. It is, therefore, extremely important to try to eliminate as much stress as possible. Ways to achieve this include:

1. Show and demonstrate the use of all equipment in the office.
2. Do not keep the patient waiting in the reception area.
3. In some cases, premedicate the patient with an antianxiety medication. This step requires a consultation with the patient's physician or neurologist.

SUMMARY

Seizures disorders are mysterious, and seizures can be frightening for both the patient and dental personnel. However, by being aware of what takes place during a seizure, members of the dental team can learn to handle this situation quickly and effectively.

REVIEW QUESTIONS

MULTIPLE CHOICE

1. If a person experiences several epileptic seizures occurring one after the other, the person is most likely experiencing
   a. an absence seizure.
   b. status epilepticus.
   c. a partial seizure.
   d. none of the above

2. In most cases epilepsy can be controlled by administering an
   a. antidepressant.
   b. anticonvulsant.
   c. antibiotic.
   d. all of the above

3. An adverse dental condition that sometimes occurs as a result of taking Dilantin is
   a. Dilantin gingival hyperplasia.
   b. Dilantin gingival atrophy.
   c. periodontosis.
   d. ANUG.

4. Which of the following is not appropriate in the treatment of an epileptic seizure?
   (1) loosen any tight clothing
   (2) restrain the patient from making any movements
   (3) remove any dental objects from the patient's mouth
   (4) do not move the patient unless it is absolutely necessary
   a. 2
   b. 3, 4
   c. 1, 2, 3, 4
   d. 4

5. Which of the following may cause a person to develop a seizure disorder?
   a. injury to the brain
   b. high fever
   c. injury during birth
   d. all the above

6. During which phase of the grand mal seizure would the tonic/clonic movements be seen?
   a. prodromal
   b. convulsive
   c. postictal
   d. none of the above

7. During what type of seizure would the patient exhibit a blank stare and twitch or blink?
   a. grand mal
   b. status epilepticus
   c. partial
   d. none of the above

8. If a person experiences an aura, it usually occurs during the _____ phase.
   a. postictal
   b. prodromal
   c. convulsive
   d. none of the above

9. Medical assistance should be summoned if
   a. status epilepticus is suspected.
   b. the patient is injured.
   c. the patient stops breathing.
   d. all the above

10. An absence or petit mal seizure is most often seen in
    a. young adults.
    b. children.
    c. elderly.
    d. all the above

TRUE OR FALSE

_____   1. All causes of epilepsy are unknown.

_____   2. A patient should not be restrained during a seizure.

_____   3. The most common type of seizure in children is a partial seizure.

_____   4. The primary goal in treating an epileptic seizure is to maintain an open airway.

_____   5. Anticonvulsants are not successful in treating most cases of epilepsy.

_____   6. Status epilepticus causes death in 10 percent of cases.

_____   7. Tonic/clonic movements are usually seen in absence (petit mal) seizures.

_____   8. It is best to use fixed dental appliances, if possible, when dealing with an epileptic.

_____   9. Dilantin gingival hyperplasia occurs in some epileptics as a result of taking Dilantin.

_____   10. Every epileptic experiences the same type of aura.

MEDICAL EMERGENCY!

CASE STUDY 5-1

A 32-year-old female presents with a positive medical history. She indicates that she has seizures that are not controlled with medication. The patient is scheduled for an initial examination. The dentist has become involved in an extensive procedure, and the patient is kept waiting in the operatory. During this time she becomes very anxious about the upcoming treatment. The dentist enters the operatory and begins treatment. The patient is very quiet and starts to twitch. She then proceeds to a full tonic-clonic seizure.

Questions

1.   What could have been done that might have prevented the patient from experiencing the seizure?

2. How would being aware that the patient has a seizure disorder help during treatment of the episode?

3. Describe the signs this patient would exhibit that would indicate the seizure was a tonic-clonic one.

4. Explain the treatment that would be provided for this patient.

CASE STUDY 5-2

PT, a 29-year-old male patient, presents with a positive medical history. He indicates that he has a seizure disorder, but has been stabilized with medications and has not had a seizure in 18 months. The dental auxiliary enters the treatment room and begins speaking to the patient about the procedure on tooth #2. As the treatment explanation continues, the patient becomes more quiet and less responsive. The auxiliary notifies the dentist of the patient's change in consciousness.

Questions

1. What type of seizure is the patient experiencing?

2. How would knowing the patient's medical history help the auxiliary know what the patient is experiencing?

3. List the steps of the treatment that would be provided for a patient experiencing a seizure.

CHAPTER 6

Diabetes Mellitus

LEARNING OUTCOMES

Upon completion of this chapter, the student will be able to:

- Define diabetes mellitus
- Explain the function of insulin
- Explain the difference between Type I and Type II diabetes
- Define oral hypoglycemics
- Explain two possible causes of diabetes
- Define hyperglycemia
- Explain the signs and symptoms of hyperglycemia
- Explain the treatment of hyperglycemia
- Define hypoglycemia
- Explain the signs and symptoms of hypoglycemia
- Define glucagon
- Explain the difference between diabetic coma and insulin shock
- Explain two medical problems associated with diabetes
- Describe one dental problem with which the diabetic patient may present

KEY TERMS

diabetic coma	HbA1C	insulin shock	neuropathy
gestational diabetes	hyperglycemia	ketones	oral hypoglycemics
glucagon	hypoglycemia	macrovascular disease	pancreas
glucose	insulin	microvascular disease	periodontal disease

The term *diabetes mellitus* came from Greek and Latin sources. Diabetes is translated as "run through a siphon"; *mellitus* means "honey." Together they are said to mean "sweet water siphon." The name *diabetes mellitus* was given to this disease because medical people of ancient times observed that persons with diabetes urinated frequently and their urine tasted very sweet. Today diabetes mellitus is defined as a disease of metabolism that occurs as a result of either a deficiency or a complete lack of insulin in the body.

HISTORY

Diabetes mellitus is certainly not a new disease; it has been reported since Roman times. However, not until the early 1920s was a lack or absence of insulin discovered to be the cause of diabetes. Around 1921, animal-obtained insulin began to be used in the treatment of diabetes. Beginning in the 1980s, technology allowed insulin to be bioengineered and produced under laboratory settings. Currently it is this type of insulin that is prescribed and used by patients with diabetes.

FUNCTIONS OF GLUCOSE AND INSULIN

glucose Fuel for the body manufactured from the food one eats.

insulin Hormone secreted by the pancreas.

pancreas Body organ that produces insulin.

neuropathy A nerve disorder that can cause numbness and sometimes pain and weakness in hands, arms, feet, and legs.

Glucose is the fuel for the body that is manufactured from the food we eat. A great many of the cells of the body must have glucose to survive. Glucose is carried to all the cells by the bloodstream. However, for glucose to be able to enter the cell and provide it with the needed fuel, **insulin** (a hormone produced in the **pancreas**) must be present. In addition, the cells must also have insulin receptors. Patients with diabetes who must take insulin have the condition in which the pancreas is either not making enough insulin or not making it at all. Patients with diabetes who do not have to take insulin have a condition in which the pancreas produces enough insulin or perhaps even too much. The problem is usually that either there are not enough insulin receptors or these receptors are defective or have a lack of sensitivity to the insulin.

It is of utmost importance that the glucose in the blood be kept at appropriate levels. Although glucose is the only fuel for the brain, it is also toxic to many tissues. Too much glucose therefore has the potential to cause as many problems as too little glucose. An imbalance of glucose in the blood results in some complications associated with diabetes, such as macrovascular disease, microvascular disease, and **neuropathy.** The imbalance also results in one of two conditions: hypoglycemia or hyperglycemia.

CAUSES

Most causes of diabetes are not definitely known, although there are some theories. First, it is known that heredity plays a definite role in causing diabetes and that diabetes is carried by one or more genes. A person may carry this gene and yet not develop the disease, but pass it on to the next generation. Therefore, if one or both parents have diabetes, the child's chances of developing diabetes are increased.

Another theory holds that Type I diabetes (see the next section on classification) may have occurred as a result of a virus related to the mumps virus that damaged the cells of the pancreas, which produces insulin.

A final theory is that Type II diabetes can occur as a result of pregnancy because pregnancy causes such a drastic change in the hormones of the body.

Other theories of the causes of diabetes are developing as more information concerning diabetes is discovered.

CLASSIFICATION

Diabetes is classified as either Type I or Type II. See Emergency Basics 6-1 for a summary of the characteristics associated with each type.

Type I diabetes was once known as "juvenile diabetes" because it usually occurs in the young. The name was changed because the condition, although not common, has occurred in older people. A Type I diabetic is insulin-dependent. This means that the body does not produce adequate insulin and the person must administer insulin on a programmed dosage set by the primary care physician. Insulin can be administered by daily injections or through an insulin pump (see Figure 6-1). Insulin cannot be taken orally because it is a protein and would be digested by the stomach. Type I diabetes accounts for a smaller percentage of all the cases of diabetes mellitus. The majority of the medical problems associated with diabetes occur in Type I, usually because the patient has diabetes for such a long time.

Type II diabetes has also been known as "adult-onset diabetes." Like Type I, this name was changed because this condition can also occur in the young. However, most people with Type II diabetes are middle-aged and obese. Type II accounts for the majority of the known cases of diabetes. In most cases of Type II, insulin is not required because the condition can usually be controlled with diet, exercise and, in some cases, oral hypoglycemics, such as sulfonylureas, thiazolidinediones, alpha-glucosidase inhibitors, and metformin.

Emergency Basics 6-1

Type I And Type II Diabetes

Type I—Insulin-Dependent Diabetes Mellitus (IDDM)
- Seen most often in the young (also known as juvenile diabetes)
- Associated most often with additional medical problems
- Requires daily insulin injections

Type II—Non-Insulin-Dependent Diabetes Mellitus (NIDDM)
- Seen most often in obese adults (also known as adult-onset diabetes)
- Usually controlled with diet and/or oral hypoglycemics
- Is increasing in younger patients due to the increased obesity levels in American society

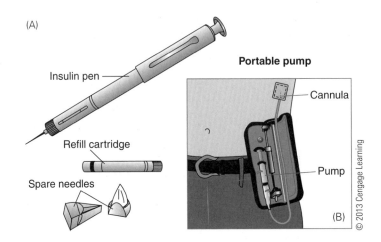

FIGURE 6-1   (A) Insulin injection pen; (B) insulin pump.

TEST YOUR KNOWLEDGE

1. What medication is IDDM treated with on a daily basis?

2. How is NIDDM treated on a daily basis?

Gestational Diabetes

gestational diabetes
Diabetes that usually occurs first during pregnancy.

An additional form of diabetes is called **gestational diabetes.** This form of diabetes begins during pregnancy and ends following delivery.

Unlike Type I diabetes, women with gestational diabetes have plenty of insulin. During pregnancy the placenta provides the developing fetus with nutrients and water from the mother. It also provides a variety of hormones that are vital to the pregnancy. Ironically, several of these hormones have a blocking effect on insulin. This blocking effect usually occurs approximately midway through the pregnancy. The larger the placenta becomes, the more blocking of the insulin occurs. This occurs in all pregnancies, and in most cases the woman is able to make additional insulin to overcome the blocking effect. However, when the pancreas makes all the insulin that it can and there still is not enough to overcome the effect of the placenta's hormones, gestational diabetes results. If the placenta's hormones from the mother's blood could be removed, the condition would end. This is what happens following delivery of the baby, and therefore gestational diabetes ends when the pregnancy ends.

Any woman may develop gestational diabetes during pregnancy. However, some women are at greater risk. Some of these risk factors are obesity; a family history of diabetes; having given birth previously to a very large infant, a stillbirth, or a child with a birth defect; or having too much amniotic fluid. Also, women who are older than 25 are at a greater risk than younger women.

The Council on Diabetes in Pregnancy of the American Diabetes Association strongly recommends that all pregnant women be screened for gestational diabetes. The most common test is the glucose-screening test.

ORAL HYPOGLYCEMICS

oral hypoglycemics Medication that can lower blood sugar.

Oral hypoglycemics are medications that lower blood sugar. They are not effective in treating Type I diabetes, in which there is no insulin production, but they have been found to be effective in some cases of Type II diabetes. Most physicians suggest that it is best to treat Type II with diet and exercise and, if medication is needed, to try oral medications. Oral hypoglycemics are not used with pregnant patients or patients with liver or kidney problems.

DIABETIC EMERGENCIES: HYPERGLYCEMIA AND HYPOGLYCEMIA

The balance of glucose in the body must remain constant. If there is too much glucose, a condition known as hyperglycemia occurs. On the other hand, if there is too little sugar, a condition known as hypoglycemia occurs. Both of these conditions have the potential to develop into an emergency situation.

Hyperglycemia

hyperglycemia A condition that occurs when there is too much glucose in the blood.

ketones Normal metabolic products from which acetone may arise spontaneously.

diabetic coma A life-threatening condition caused by a lack of insulin in the body.

Hyperglycemia occurs when there is too much glucose (sugar) in the blood and is usually seen when there is a deficiency or complete lack of insulin. Hyperglycemia is a slow-occurring condition. A person with hyperglycemia exhibits increased thirst and urination. Because of the imbalance created in the cells, there is dehydration, which results in the increased thirst and ultimately increased urination. If the urine is checked, there will be a large amount of sugar and **ketones.** The patient may also exhibit loss of appetite, nausea and/or vomiting, fatigue, abdominal pains, and generalized aches. If the condition is allowed to progress, the patient exhibits a heavy, labored breathing called Kussmaul breathing. The patient's breath has a fruity acetone odor as a result of the extra sugar. This is the condition present in the undiagnosed diabetic patient. Without treatment, this person will lose consciousness, going into what is called a **diabetic coma,** and die.

Diabetic coma was the most common cause of death among people with diabetes in the years before the discovery of insulin. Today diabetic coma should rarely occur in known diabetic patients because its symptoms are identifiable for several days before the coma occurs. Also, if the diabetic patient is testing the blood sugar on a regular basis using a glucometer (see Figure 6-2), the patient will be able to identify problems before they advance as far as diabetic coma. Diabetic coma can nevertheless cause death to patients with diabetes, especially patients with uncontrolled diabetes.

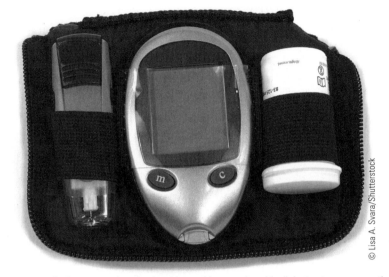

FIGURE 6-2   A glucometer is a testing kit used by people with diabetes to measure the level of sugar in blood.

People who experience hyperglycemia require insulin injections; if conscious, they should administer their own insulin. Patients who are unconscious and experiencing a diabetic coma should be transported to a medical facility by the emergency medical service. The dental staff should never attempt to administer insulin to an unconscious patient because the amount of insulin required is not known.

See Emergency Basics 6-2 for a summary of the signs and treatment of hyperglycemia.

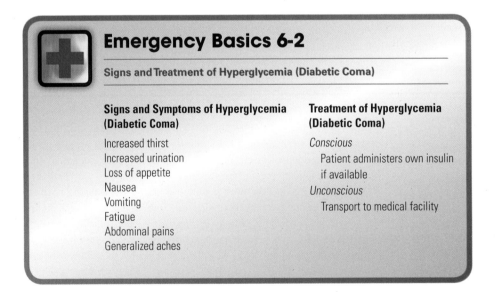

Emergency Basics 6-2

Signs and Treatment of Hyperglycemia (Diabetic Coma)

Signs and Symptoms of Hyperglycemia (Diabetic Coma)

Increased thirst
Increased urination
Loss of appetite
Nausea
Vomiting
Fatigue
Abdominal pains
Generalized aches

Treatment of Hyperglycemia (Diabetic Coma)

Conscious
   Patient administers own insulin if available
Unconscious
   Transport to medical facility

Hypoglycemia

hypoglycemia
A condition that occurs as a result of too little glucose in the body.

insulin shock
A life-threatening condition caused by an excess of insulin in the body.

Hypoglycemia, also known as **insulin shock,** occurs as a result of too little glucose in the body. Since glucose is the only source of fuel for the brain, if the brain goes for a long time without adequate glucose, brain-cell damage may occur.

Hypoglycemia usually has a rapid onset and may be caused by any of the following situations:

1. The diabetic patient may have skipped a meal or not eaten the balanced diet their disease requires. As a result, the insulin level is too high and the glucose level too low. Important questions to ask patients who have diabetes prior to any dental treatment are when they ate their last meal and what they ate. The answers to these questions can help the dental auxiliary determine whether or not a diabetic emergency is possible.

2. For some reason, the patient may have experienced an unusual amount of exercise, which burned up the sugar sources within the body. Diabetic patients are encouraged to exercise. As a matter of fact, several famous athletes have diabetes. However, there must always be a constant balance among exercise, food, and insulin. Diabetic patients monitor their blood glucose levels with multiple checks throughout the day and night.

3. A change in routine occurs, such as when a young person goes off to college. The new patterns, schedules, and emotional stress may all cause an imbalance in the insulin and glucose levels that may result in hypoglycemia.

A person exhibiting hypoglycemia may break out in a cold sweat and appear nervous, trembling, weak, and hungry. There is usually a personality change that may include irritability, confusion, and the inability to think clearly. Often a family member or close associate of the patient may be better able to detect warning signs of hypoglycemia than the patient, since the patient may be confused. Sometimes the patient may become upset and refuse treatment as a result of confusion.

This patient requires treatment as soon as possible. Treatment for hypoglycemia includes getting some type of sugar source into the patient's system. If the patient is conscious, the easiest method is to give a glass of orange juice, although any fast-acting glucose source will help. Examples of fast-acting glucose sources are: 8 ounces of milk, ½ teaspoon of honey or cake icing, 4 ounces of regular (not diet) soda. Some companies are now manufacturing a liquid sugar source that is available in a tube and is easy to administer to the patient. If the patient is unconscious, do not attempt to give anything by mouth. Instead, the person should be treated with an injection of glucagon.

glucagon
A hormone produced in the pancreas that raises blood sugar.

Glucagon is a hormone, produced in the pancreas, that raises blood sugar. It achieves this effect by changing the sugar stored in the liver into a source of sugar that can be used by the body. As soon as hypoglycemia is diagnosed in the unconscious patient, an injection of glucagon should be given. Once the patient regains full consciousness, orange juice should be administered. Glucagon is used up very quickly, and if another source of sugar is not given, the patient may relapse into hypoglycemia.

See Emergency Basics 6-3 for a summary of the signs and treatment of hypoglycemia.

Emergency Basics 6-3

Signs and Treatment of Hypoglycemia (Insulin Shock)

Signs and Symptoms of Hypoglycemia (Insulin Shock)	Treatment of Hypoglycemia (Insulin Shock)
Cold sweat	*Conscious*
Nervousness	Administer sugar source
Trembling	*Unconscious*
Weakness	Give injection of glucagon
Hunger	Administer sugar source
Personality change	
Confusion	

TEST YOUR KNOWLEDGE

1. What are the noticeable signs and symptoms of hypoglycemia?

2. What can occur if the patient is not treated for hypoglycemia?

Diabetic Coma or Insulin Shock?

If the dental team finds a diabetic patient unconscious, it will be hard to determine whether the patient is experiencing a diabetic coma, insulin shock, or a related medical problem. If the dental team knows from the patient's medical history that the patient has Type II diabetes and does not self-administer insulin, they may infer that the patient is experiencing a diabetic coma and should receive immediate medical attention. If the team members have no idea what type of diabetes the patient has, then they should treat the condition as insulin shock. It is very important to get glucose into the system before the brain is damaged. An individual can withstand very high levels of blood sugar much longer than the brain can survive with low levels of glucose. Therefore, if the dental team does not know which condition the patient is experiencing, they should treat for insulin shock. Once this treatment is performed, if recovery does not occur, the team should summon medical help.

MEDICAL PROBLEMS

macrovascular disease Disease of the large vessels of the body.

microvascular disease Disease of the small vessels of the body.

In addition to hypoglycemia and hyperglycemia, diabetic patients also have an increased risk of other medical problems. Diabetes increases the risk of **macrovascular** (large-vessel) and **microvascular** (small-vessel) abnormalities.

Large-vessel problems are indicated by:

1. inadequate blood supply to the heart muscle, resulting in conditions such as myocardial infarction or angina pectoris
2. inadequate blood supply to the brain, resulting in various types of cerebrovascular accidents
3. inadequate blood supply to the legs, which increases the risk of infection and tissue necrosis
4. inadequate blood supply to the kidneys, which results in kidney dysfunction or failure

Small-vessel problems most often affect the small vessels of the eye. This causes a disease known as diabetic retinopathy. This disease can cause blindness in patients with diabetes.

See Emergency Basics 6-4 for a summary of common medical problems associated with diabetes.

Emergency Basics 6-4

Common Medical Problems Associated with Diabetes

Macrovascular
- Myocardial infarction (see Chapter 11)
- Angina pectoris (see Chapter 11)
- High blood pressure
- Cerebrovascular accident (see Chapter 7)
- Tissue necrosis
- Kidney dysfunction

Microvascular
- Diabetic retinopathy

ORAL MANIFESTATIONS

The diabetic dental patient can present some unique problems for both dentist and dental staff. First there is the strong possibility that the patient may experience diabetic coma or insulin shock while in the office—the emotional stress of experiencing a dental procedure may be enough to exacerbate an already unstable situation.

If the patient is experiencing a particular medical problem associated with diabetes, such as high blood pressure or cardiovascular disease, the dental team may have to alter its treatment to avoid an emergency situation.

In addition, the diabetic patient may experience some specific dental problems. For example, **periodontal disease** is extremely common in patients with diabetes. Furthermore, the periodontal disease tends to be very severe and hard to control no matter how well the patient maintains good oral hygiene. There have been situations in which severe periodontal disease has caused a person's diabetes to become uncontrolled due to the level of infection and inflammation. Therefore the importance of keeping the periodontal disease to a minimum can be easily seen, and this can sometimes be achieved through good oral hygiene.

Patients with diabetes sometimes have problems healing and are very prone to infection. This is a result of the circulatory problems associated with macrovascular and microvascular disease. The dental team, therefore, needs to be very careful and cause as little tissue trauma as possible. Furthermore, if dental surgery is performed, extra appointments should be made on a frequent basis to make sure the patient is healing properly.

When treating a dental patient with diabetes, the dental team should ensure the following:

1. Maintain a current, thorough medical history. It is important to realize the patient has diabetes. It is also important to know whether the patient is Type I or Type II and if the condition is controlled or uncontrolled at the time of the dental appointment.

2. Consult with the patient's physician before beginning any extensive treatment. If the treatment that is to be provided will interfere with maintaining a normal routine, the patient's physician may need to make some changes in the insulin dose. There may also be some underlying medical problems that require special treatment or medication. It may be necessary to evaluate the patient's last **HbA1C** to determine how well controlled the patient's disease has been.

3. Attempt to keep the patient calm and relaxed during all phases of treatment. As previously mentioned, emotional stress or upset can trigger particular medical problems in the patient with diabetes.

4. Avoid making appointments that would cause the patient to miss a scheduled meal. Keeping diabetes under control means maintaining a balance among food, insulin, and exercise. Scheduling an appointment during lunch, for example, may upset the insulin balance and perhaps cause the patient to experience insulin shock. It may be necessary to monitor the patient's blood glucose levels using the patient's glucometer, especially if an appointment has interfered with a scheduled meal or snack.

It is very beneficial for the members of the dental team to familiarize themselves with characteristics associated with diabetes. This is extremely helpful when providing treatment to certain age groups and patients with diabetes. For example, children with diabetes are sometimes concerned about experiencing new situations such as a trip to the dental office because they feel the dental staff will not understand their diabetes and therefore will not know what to do if they have any problems. It is important for each

periodontal disease Disease of the periodontium.

HbA1C A lab test that shows the average amount of glucose in blood over a three-month period.

member of the team to understand the disease not just to know how to treat an emergency but also to know how to talk to and work with the patient.

In addition, adolescents may present the dental team with emergency problems, because at this stage they tend to be very rebellious and may not be monitoring and controlling their diabetes as they should. Therefore, those whose diabetes is not controlled may experience a reaction while receiving dental treatment.

SUMMARY

The study and treatment of diabetes has been focused for only about 60 years; advancements are being made rather rapidly and have been remarkable. New methods of diagnosing, treating, and controlling diabetes have been discovered. The space program has resulted in several advancements in the treatment of diabetes. Hopefully, in the near future, advancements will be made that will mean the dental team may not have to deal with emergencies such as diabetic coma and insulin shock.

REVIEW QUESTIONS

MULTIPLE CHOICE

1. Type I diabetes is most often treated with daily injections of
   a. glucagon.
   b. insulin.
   c. oral hypoglycemics.
   d. glucose.

2. Type II diabetes may sometimes be treated with
   a. oral hypoglycemics.
   b. glucagon.
   c. glucose.
   d. none of the above

3. Which of the following are signs or symptoms of hyperglycemia?
   (1) increased thirst
   (2) Kussmaul breathing
   (3) confusion
   (4) increased urination
   a. 1, 2, 3, 4
   b. 1, 2, 3
   c. 1, 2, 4
   d. 2, 3, 4

4. Diabetic coma is treated with
   a. glucagon.
   b. glucose.
   c. insulin.
   d. none of the above

5. Which of the following are not signs or symptoms of insulin shock?
   (1) rapid onset
   (2) cold sweat
   (3) confusion
   (4) increased thirst
   a. 1, 2
   b. 3, 4
   c. 1
   d. 4

6. The unconscious patient suffering from insulin shock should be treated by
   a. giving orange juice.
   b. administering insulin injection.
   c. administering oral hypoglycemics.
   d. administering a glucagon injection.

7. An example of a microvascular disease is
   a. angina pectoris.
   b. diabetic retinopathy.
   c. kidney dysfunction.
   d. cerebrovascular accident.

8. The only fuel for the brain is
   a. glucose.
   b. insulin.
   c. glucagon.
   d. none of the above

9. The correct treatment for the conscious patient suffering from insulin shock is to
   a. administer a sugar source such as orange juice.
   b. administer insulin.
   c. administer a glucagon injection.
   d. none of the above

10. A dental patient with diabetes may be more prone to
    a. decay.
    b. periodontal disease.
    c. malocclusion.
    d. all the above

TRUE OR FALSE

————————   1. Insulin may not be taken orally because it is digested by the stomach.

————————   2. Most medical problems are associated with Type II diabetes.

————————   3. Diabetic coma was the leading cause of death among patients with diabetes before the discovery of insulin.

————————   4. Type II diabetes was once called juvenile diabetes.

————————   5. Diabetes is a disease that originated in the early 1900s.

————————   6. Type II diabetes accounts for the majority of the diagnosed cases of diabetes.

————————   7. Type I diabetes can usually be controlled with diet.

————————   8. Heredity plays an important part in the cause of diabetes.

————————   9. Insulin is produced in the body by the pancreas.

————————   10. Hypoglycemia results when there is too much sugar in the bloodstream.

MEDICAL EMERGENCY!

CASE STUDY 6-1

A 35-year-old female presents with a positive medical history. She is an insulin-dependent diabetic. Her treatment for today is an amalgam restoration. The dental auxiliary reviews the medical history and finds that the patient is a Type I diabetic taking daily injections of insulin. The patient rushes into the office slightly late for her appointment. She reports that she was in such a hurry that she did not get a chance to eat lunch. As the appointment begins, she breaks out in a cold sweat and appears very nervous. When the dentist questions her, she seems confused.

Questions

1.   What condition is the patient most likely experiencing?

2.   What should be done to treat this condition?

3.   How might this situation have been avoided?

CASE STUDY 6-2

A 23-year-old female presents with a positive medical history. She reports a history of Type I diabetes. The patient is scheduled for a crown preparation at the noon hour. When the dental auxiliary reviews the medical history, the patient indicates that she has an insulin pump. As the treatment progresses, the dental auxiliary notices that the patient's skin has become cold and clammy, and when the patient is questioned, she appears to be very confused.

Questions

1.   What type of diabetes does the patient have?

2.   What condition is the patient most likely experiencing?

3.   How could this episode have been avoided?

CHAPTER 7

Cerebrovascular Accident (CVA)

LEARNING OUTCOMES

Upon completion of this chapter, the student will be able to:

- Define cerebrovascular accident (CVA)
- List the predisposing factors of a CVA
- Define the different classifications of a CVA
- List the signs and symptoms of a CVA
- Describe the treatment of a CVA

KEY TERMS

aneurysm	cranium	hemiplegia	ischemia
atherosclerosis	edema	hemorrhage	lumen
cerebral infarction	embolism	hypertension	thrombosis

A cerebrovascular accident, also known as a CVA or stroke, is defined as a specific neu-rologic deficit that occurs suddenly as a result of vascular disease of a hemorrhagic or ischemic nature (Figure 7-1). The extent of the deficit depends on both the area of the brain involved and the cause of the deficit.

CLASSIFICATIONS

Cerebrovascular accidents are classified according to cause. The causes of CVAs can be divided into the following categories: cerebral embolism, cerebral infarction, cerebral hemorrhage, and cerebral thrombosis. The signs and symptoms associated with each cause are similar, as is the treatment. Each type is discussed separately. Figure 7-2 shows an MRI of a CVA.

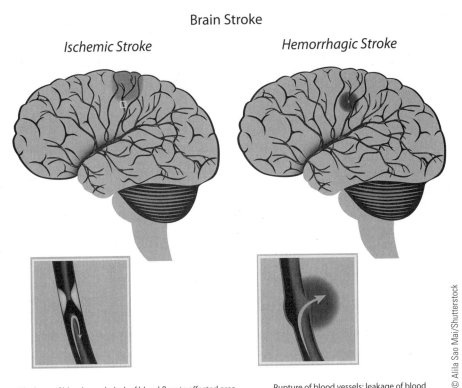

Brain Stroke

Ischemic Stroke   *Hemorrhagic Stroke*

Blockage of blood vessels; lack of blood flow to affected area   Rupture of blood vessels; leakage of blood

© Alila Sao Mai/Shutterstock

FIGURE 7-1   An ischemic stroke (left) happens when there is a sudden blockage, usually caused by a blood clot that deprives areas of the brain of proper oxygen. Ischemic strokes are the most common. A hemorrhagic stroke (right) is the rupturing of a blood vessel, resulting in a dramatic decrease in blood flow to the brain. An infarct is an area in the brain tissue that has died due to a lack of blood.

embolism A clot that forms somewhere in the body and travels throughout the body until it lodges in a smaller vessel.

hemorrhage A large amount of blood loss in a short period of time.

cranium The part of the skull that houses the brain.

edema Local or generalized swelling from retention of excessive fluid.

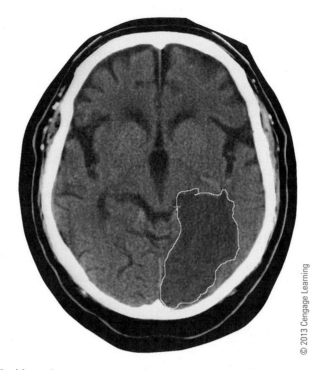

© 2013 Cengage Learning

FIGURE 7-2   Magnetic resonance image of a brain with a visible bleed from a CVA in the lower-right section of the brain.

CEREBRAL EMBOLISM

A cerebral **embolism** is a stroke that occurs as a result of a wandering clot or embolus that may become lodged in a cerebral artery and thus reduce or cut off the blood supply to the area of the brain beyond the clot. In practically all cerebral embolisms, the clot begins in the heart, aorta, or other proximal large vessel.

The cerebral deficit associated with the embolism usually occurs very rapidly. The damage is worst at the beginning and usually does not increase in severity. However, there may be quick improvement in some patients because the embolus may dissolve or break up.

A cerebral embolism occurs most often in patients who are awake. A mild headache is usually the first symptom, with the other neurological signs and symptoms associated with a CVA following within several hours.

CEREBRAL HEMORRHAGE

A cerebral **hemorrhage** occurs when an artery ruptures and fills the **cranium** with blood, resulting in an increase in the pressure within the cranium. This increase in pressure can cause a displacement of the brain and ultimately death. Cerebral **edema**, swelling of the neural tissue, always develops and adds to the high death rate from this type of CVA.

The two main sources of cerebral hemorrhage are a ruptured **aneurysm** and hypertensive vascular disease. The rupture in both these cases usually occurs as a result of an abrupt change in systolic blood pressure. The stress and anxiety associated with various dental procedures can cause this rise in systolic pressure.

Although cerebral hemorrhage is seen most often in older patients, it may also occur in young patients as a result of a ruptured aneurysm or malformed blood vessel.

A cerebral hemorrhage usually occurs when the patient is awake and active, so it is not uncommon for this type of CVA to occur in the dental office.

Signs and symptoms may appear very quickly and then increase in severity over a short period of time. Victims of a hemorrhage often complain of an excruciating headache. The headache is localized at first, but as the bleeding spreads, the headache also spreads. The headache associated with a hemorrhage occurs because the blood has an irritating effect on the neural tissues.

Other signs and symptoms include nausea and vomiting, chills and sweating, and dizziness. Severe neurologic deficit such as **hemiplegia** or coma may occur. The severity of the symptoms is usually related to the amount of intracranial bleeding.

On the average, one-third of these patients lose consciousness within a few minutes of onset. This indicates that a large hemorrhage has occurred, and usually there is a poor prognosis.

CEREBRAL INFARCTION

Cerebral infarction is a type of CVA that occurs as a result of some problem in the arterial blood supply from the heart to the brain. This problem usually occurs as a result of **atherosclerosis.** In these cases there is a thickening in the wall of an artery due to fatty deposits adhering to the wall (see Figure 7-3). The thickening causes a reduction in the size of the artery's **lumen,** which causes a decrease in the amount of oxygenated blood going to a particular area of the brain.

Cross sections through a coronary artery undergoing
progressive atherosclerosis and arteriosclerosis

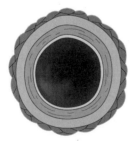
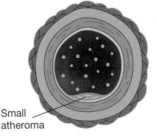
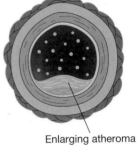

Normal artery with
open lumen

Small
atheroma

Elevated cholesterol
and blood fats

Enlarging atheroma
(plaque deposit)

© 2013 Cengage Learning

FIGURE 7-3   Progression of coronary artery disease, a risk factor for a cerebrovascular accident.

lumen The cavity of a tubular organ such as a blood vessel.

Since this type of stroke is slow in developing, noticeable neurologic deficits are also slow in developing. Unlike most classes of CVAs, headache, nausea, and vomiting are usually not present. Furthermore, the patient usually awakens in the morning with neurologic deficits from the **ischemia** that occurred during the night.

CEREBRAL THROMBOSIS

ischemia Deficiency of blood supply.

The last main cause of CVA is a cerebral **thrombosis,** which occurs when there is an obstruction of the cerebral artery by a clot that forms within that artery. This differs from an embolism, in which the clot forms in another area of the body.

thrombosis A clot that forms in a vessel.

Atherosclerosis is also a main cause of cerebral thrombosis. To prevent cerebral thrombosis, it is extremely important to aggressively treat conditions associated with atherosclerosis such as **hypertension.**

Like cerebral infarction, thrombosis very commonly happens during sleep and the patient awakens with the resulting signs of a stroke. Signs such as stuttering or other gradual deficits that reach their maximum in one to three days are often associated with thrombosis.

TRANSIENT ISCHEMIC ATTACK

hypertension Abnormally high pressure of the blood against the arterial walls; commonly known as *high blood pressure.*

A transient ischemic attack (TIA) is a neurologic deficit that lasts for a short period of time. Although a TIA is not an actual stroke, it is included in the classification of a CVA because it is so similar. The relationship between a TIA and a CVA is very similar to that of angina and myocardial infarction discussed in Chapter 11. It has been found through careful questioning of patients who have experienced a stroke that they usually experienced some episodes of TIA before they experienced the complete cerebrovascular accident.

Sometimes it is difficult to determine whether the patient is suffering from a CVA or from a TIA. The best way to make that determination is by the duration of the episode. The TIA lasts only a few minutes and then the signs and symptoms cease, whereas the signs and symptoms of a true CVA do not regress.

The clinical manifestations of a TIA vary according to the area of the brain affected. However, most people suffering from a TIA experience some numbness or weakness in the extremities. This numbness is sometimes described by the patient as a "pins-and-needles" feeling. Consciousness is usually not impaired, but the patient may appear somewhat confused during the episode.

The TIA does not usually present an emergency situation in the dental office. However, if the patient has a history of repeated TIAs, the dental team should realize that this patient has increased chances for experiencing a severe CVA.

Always remember that a TIA has the potential to advance to a severe CVA. Whether a TIA advances to a complete stroke usually depends on the underlying cause of the TIA. If the cause is resolved, a complete stroke will not occur.

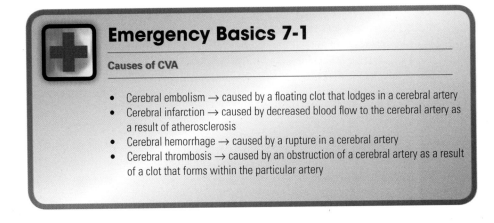

Emergency Basics 7-1

Causes of CVA

- Cerebral embolism → caused by a floating clot that lodges in a cerebral artery
- Cerebral infarction → caused by decreased blood flow to the cerebral artery as a result of atherosclerosis
- Cerebral hemorrhage → caused by a rupture in a cerebral artery
- Cerebral thrombosis → caused by an obstruction of a cerebral artery as a result of a clot that forms within the particular artery

See Emergency Basics 7-1 for a summary of the various causes of CVA. Although it is beneficial for the dental auxiliary to understand these causes, it is not necessary to distinguish between them to provide proper emergency treatment. Emergency treatment in the dental setting is basically the same for any CVA, regardless of the cause.

TEST YOUR KNOWLEDGE

1. What type of stroke is a result of a clot forming in some area of the body and traveling to the brain?

2. What type of stroke is most likely to occur in the dental office?

3. What type of stroke is a CVA with signs and symptoms that are exhibited for only a few minutes?

SIGNS AND SYMPTOMS

Signs and symptoms of a CVA vary, depending on the area affected and the type of CVA. Specific signs and symptoms of the various causes of a CVA have been covered; however, some similar signs and symptoms that are usually seen when a dental patient experiences a CVA are:

1. Headache may be the first symptom in several types, but other neurological signs and symptoms will soon develop.
2. Unconsciousness may occur. This is usually an ominous sign and indicates a severe stroke.

3. Paralysis may occur in the extremities of both sides, although most often it is unilateral.
4. Conscious patients may appear confused and have difficulty in understanding where they are or what has happened.
5. Speech is usually impaired as a result of paralysis in some of the facial muscles or in the areas of the brain associated with speech.
6. The pupils of the eyes are usually of unequal size, a sign evident in both the conscious and unconscious patient.
7. The patient may experience difficulty in breathing.

See Emergency Basics 7-2 for a summary of the signs and symptoms of CVA.

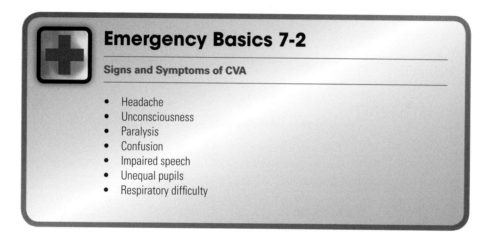

Emergency Basics 7-2

Signs and Symptoms of CVA

- Headache
- Unconsciousness
- Paralysis
- Confusion
- Impaired speech
- Unequal pupils
- Respiratory difficulty

The American Red Cross teaches a mnemonic in its First Aid course that can be used to determine very quickly whether a patient may be experiencing the signs and symptoms of a cerebrovascular accident. The mnemonic is FAST. See Emergency Basics 7-3.

Emergency Basics 7-3

Recognizing a CVA: FAST

- **F = FACE** Ask the patient to smile. An asymmetry or drooping of one side of the face can indicate a potential stroke.
- **A = ARM** Ask the patient to lift both arms. A weakness of one arm or inability to raise an arm can indicate a potential stroke.
- **S = SPEECH** Ask the patient to repeat a simple statement. Evaluate both the patient's ability to respond correctly and the patient's speech pattern (e.g., whether the phrasing is correct and whether speech is slurred).
- **T = TIME** Notify the dentist and activate the emergency protocols in the office as quickly as possible. Noting the time and extent of the deficits can be helpful to the responding emergency personnel.

TEST YOUR KNOWLEDGE

1. What medical conditions on a patient's medical history indicate that the patient might have an increased risk of experiencing a CVA?

2. What are the general signs and symptoms of a CVA?

3. What are the signs and symptoms associated with a cerebral hemorrhage?

TREATMENT

If a CVA occurs while the patient is in the dental office, the dental team should not waste time trying to determine the cause. The same emergency treatment is administered regardless of cause.

A dental team that recognizes the signs and symptoms of a CVA should be most concerned with monitoring the patient's respiratory and circulatory status. It is important to make sure the airway is open and adequate oxygen is available, since the patient is already suffering from an oxygen deficiency.

Specifically, treatment for a CVA should include:

1. Stop all dental treatment. Make sure to remove all objects from in and around the patient's mouth.
2. Position the patient with the head slightly elevated to relieve intracranial pressure.
3. Monitor the vital signs. This will provide helpful information for the paramedic unit.
4. Administer oxygen. The patient is suffering from an oxygen deficiency, so this helps to make the patient more comfortable.
5. Summon medical assistance. This patient requires more extensive treatment than the dental team is able to provide. It is of utmost importance that the patient be transported to a medical facility as soon as possible.
6. Keep the patient calm and quiet. It is important that the patient not become overheated or upset, since this can hasten brain damage.
7. Be prepared to provide basic life support. At any point it may become necessary to perform CPR, and the dental team should be prepared for this at all times.
8. Avoid giving any medication to the patient that could affect the emergency room physician's ability to determine changes in neurological status.

See Emergency Basics 7-4 for a summary of the treatment of CVA.

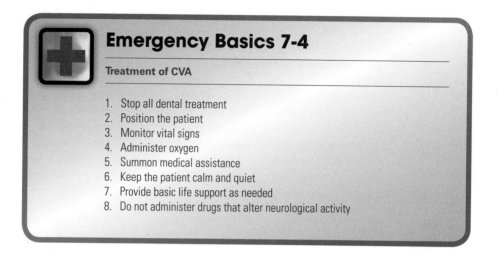

Emergency Basics 7-4

Treatment of CVA

1. Stop all dental treatment
2. Position the patient
3. Monitor vital signs
4. Administer oxygen
5. Summon medical assistance
6. Keep the patient calm and quiet
7. Provide basic life support as needed
8. Do not administer drugs that alter neurological activity

Any time the dental team deals with someone who has experienced a CVA, it must keep in mind that the person may die at any time; resuscitation efforts will not help because there has been extensive brain damage. Nevertheless, if it becomes necessary, the dental team must always attempt to resuscitate the patient.

Furthermore, even though CVA patients may not be able to speak, if they are conscious they are probably able to hear everything that is said, so the dental team must be very careful not to say anything that might upset the patient.

TEST YOUR KNOWLEDGE

1. Why would you not position the patient experiencing a CVA in the Trendelenburg position?

2. What effect would administering pain medication have on a patient's treatment at the hospital?

3. Why should EMS be called as soon as possible when a dental patient is experiencing the signs and symptoms of a CVA?

SUMMARY

Fortunately, a CVA is not a common occurrence in the dental office. Nevertheless, it can occur and therefore the dental team must be prepared to treat such patients. As with all emergencies, the best treatment is prevention. The dental team can best achieve this by realizing that certain people are prone to CVAs. For example, diabetics, those suffering from hypertension, those with a history of cardiac disease, and those with a history of TIAs are more likely than other patients to experience a CVA in the dental office.

Furthermore, people who survive a CVA are at a high risk of recurrence. If the dental team is treating a post-CVA patient or a patient at risk for experiencing a first-time CVA, extreme care must be taken to control anxiety and pain, which could easily trigger a CVA. The CVA presents a difficult emergency for the dental team. It is best to do everything possible to prevent a CVA and to be totally prepared to provide the best treatment possible should one occur.

REVIEW QUESTIONS

MULTIPLE CHOICE

1. A stroke in which signs and symptoms are exhibited for only a few minutes is known as a
   a. RIND.
   b. cerebral embolism.
   c. cerebral infarction.
   d. none of the above

2. A stroke that occurs as a result of a clot forming in some area of the body and traveling to the brain is known as a
   a. cerebral infarction.
   b. cerebral embolism.
   c. cerebral thrombosis.
   d. TIA.

3. What type of stroke is most likely to occur in the dental office?
   a. cerebral hemorrhage
   b. cerebral embolism
   c. cerebral infarction
   d. all the above

4. Which of the following conditions may result in a cerebral hemorrhage?
   (1) aneurysm
   (2) emboli
   (3) hypertensive vascular disease
   (4) ischemia
     a. 1, 2, 3
     b. 1, 3, 4
     c. 1, 2

5. Cerebral thrombosis occurs most often as a result of
     a. atherosclerosis.
     b. aneurysm.
     c. embolism.
     d. none of the above

6. A patient suffering from a stroke should be positioned
     a. in the Trendelenburg position.
     b. in the supine position.
     c. upright.
     d. with the head slightly elevated.

7. Which of the following patients have increased chances of experiencing a CVA?
   (1) hypertensive
   (2) diabetic
   (3) history of heart disease
   (4) history of TIA
     a. 1, 2, 3
     b. 2, 3
     c. 1, 4
     d. 1, 2, 3, 4

8. Which of the following are signs or symptoms of a CVA?
   (1) headache
   (2) paralysis
   (3) nausea
   (4) dizziness
     a. 1, 2
     b. 1, 2, 3
     c. 2, 4
     d. 1, 2, 3, 4

9. Which of the following is/are included in the emergency treatment of a CVA?
   (1) administer a CNS relaxer
   (2) maintain an open airway
   (3) administer oxygen
   (4) summon medical assistance
   a. 1, 2, 3, 4
   b. 1, 2, 4
   c. 2, 3, 4
   d. 1, 3, 4

10. Signs and symptoms associated with a cerebral hemorrhage include
   (1) vertigo.
   (2) vomiting.
   (3) stupor.
   (4) difficulty in movement.
   a. 1, 3, 4
   b. 4
   c. 1, 2, 3, 4
   d. 2, 3

TRUE OR FALSE

_____   1. TIAs usually last at least 48 hours.

_____   2. Cerebral embolisms usually occur while the patient is awake.

_____   3. A cerebral hemorrhage is usually preceded by a headache.

_____   4. A cerebral thrombosis occurs as a result of an obstruction of the cerebral artery by a clot that forms within the artery.

_____   5. It is imperative that the dental team know what caused the CVA before it can provide proper treatment.

_____   6. Paralysis associated with a CVA is usually unilateral.

_____   7. Signs and symptoms of a CVA vary according to the area of the brain affected as well as the type of CVA.

_____   8. People who survive a CVA experience a low risk of recurrence.

_____   9. Anxiety and pain associated with a dental appointment have the potential to trigger a CVA.

_____   10. It is uncommon for a patient to experience a TIA prior to experiencing a severe stroke.

MEDICAL EMERGENCY!

CASE STUDY 7-1

A 45-year-old male presents with a positive medical history. He documents on the health history that he is being treated by a physician for hypertension. At the current time his blood pressure is within normal range for his age and gender. While in the office he loses consciousness, then regains consciousness but is unable to speak. The dentist determines that the patient is experiencing a CVA.

Questions

1. State the signs and symptoms of a CVA.

2. Why is the patient's physician's diagnosis an important observation for the dental team to note?

3. State the treatment that will be performed for this patient.

CASE STUDY 7-2

A 65-year-old female presents with a positive medical history. She states that she has had six documented TIAs within the last twelve months. She is in the dental office for the extraction of the maxillary third molars. She states to the dental auxiliary that she is very anxious and was unable to sleep the night before due to anxiety. Before the dentist can enter the treatment room the patient loses consciousness.

Questions

1. What specific CVA is the patient experiencing?

2. Why is this condition the most common CVA that can occur in the dental office?

3. State the treatment that would be administered to this patient.

SECTION THREE

Respiratory Distress Emergencies

This section deals with medical conditions and emergencies that involve the respiratory system.

CHAPTER 8:   Asthma
CHAPTER 9:   Hyperventilation
CHAPTER 10: Airway Obstruction

CHAPTER 8

Asthma

LEARNING OUTCOMES

Upon completion of this chapter, the student will be able to:

- Define asthma
- Explain two of the causes of asthma
- Describe the signs and symptoms of asthma
- Describe the treatment provided for an asthma attack

KEY TERMS

allergen	epinephrine	intrinsic asthma	tracheobronchial tree
bronchodilator	extrinsic asthma	status asthmaticus	

**tracheobron-
chial tree** The
trachea, bronchi,
and the bronchial
tubes.

**extrinsic
asthma** A
form of asthma
caused by the
exposure of
the bronchial
mucosa to an
inhaled airborne
antigen.

Diseases or problems associated with the respiratory system such as asthma, bronchitis, or emphysema may create emergency situations. An asthma attack is one example of a respiratory emergency commonly seen in the dental setting.

Asthma is a disease of the respiratory tract that can affect all aspects of the **tracheobronchial tree:** trachea, bronchi, and bronchioles (see Figure 8-1 for an illustration). The type of asthma as well as its severity determine what areas of the tracheobronchial tree are involved. Asthma can result in the death of a patient, but currently death from asthma is a rare occurrence. Asthma affects a large percentage of the population and is not selective as to ethnicity, gender, or age.

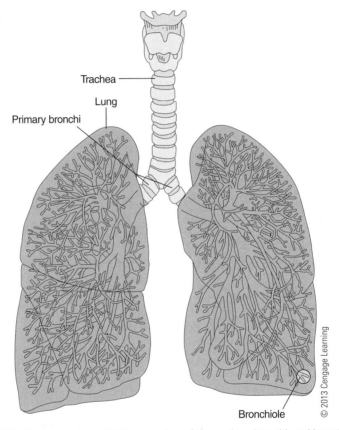

Trachea

Lung

Primary bronchi

Bronchiole

© 2013 Cengage Learning

FIGURE 8-1   The tracheobronchial tree consists of the trachea, bronchi, and bronchioles. Asthma affects all aspects of the tracheobronchial tree because it's a respiratory disease.

TYPES

Asthma can be divided into different categories. The first is **extrinsic asthma,** or allergic asthma. This type of asthma is reported most often in children and young adults. Episodes of extrinsic asthma usually result from exposure to an **allergen** such as dust,

allergen Any substance capable of inducing an allergic reaction.

pollen, animals, and certain foods and many other substances. In addition this type of asthma can be classified as exercise-induced. Most patients are aware of the types of allergens or conditions that trigger their asthma attacks and try to avoid them. If the allergens are not known, they can be determined by a physician performing allergy tests. The dental team should also be aware of any specific allergens that trigger a patient's asthma in order to avoid exposing the patient to them while the patient is in the office. See Emergency Basics 8-1 for a list of common allergens found in a dental office.

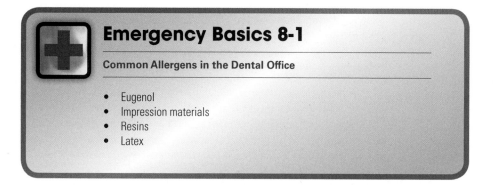

Emergency Basics 8-1

Common Allergens in the Dental Office

- Eugenol
- Impression materials
- Resins
- Latex

intrinsic asthma A nonallergic form of asthma usually first occurring later in life that tends to be chronic and persistent rather than episodic.

status asthmaticus A severe form of asthma in which the victim experiences a continuous asthma attack.

The extrinsic asthmatic patient usually does not exhibit any signs or symptoms of asthma between episodes. Furthermore, extrinsic asthma usually responds well to medication and *may* be outgrown.

A second type of asthma is **intrinsic asthma,** or infectious asthma, most often seen in patients older than age 35. Intrinsic asthma usually occurs as a result of some type of bronchial infection. Unlike the extrinsic asthma patient, this patient may exhibit a chronic cough with sputum production between attacks.

The most severe form of asthma is **status asthmaticus,** which can occur in any type of asthma. It will not respond to normal drug therapy and will cause death if not treated promptly.

TEST YOUR KNOWLEDGE

1. What type of asthma is considered the most life-threatening?

2. What type of asthma is usually reported in young children?

3. What type of asthma usually occurs as a result of a bronchial infection?

A patient may experience extrinsic or intrinsic asthma independently, or may experience a combination of the two.

CAUSES

Asthma attacks can be triggered by an almost endless number of causes, both known and unknown. As previously mentioned, exposure to a particular allergen can cause an attack. Anxiety or emotional upset is definitely known to be a factor in triggering asthma attacks—and is the main cause of asthma attacks in the dental office. Some children experience an asthma attack immediately upon entering the dental operatory, one that ends as soon as the child is removed from the operatory. It is extremely important for the dental staff to do everything possible to prevent emotional upsets by taking the following measures:

1. Do not keep the patient waiting for an extended period.
2. Explain and demonstrate the procedures and equipment.
3. Do not use threatening terminology such as *drill, hurt,* and *shot.*

TEST YOUR KNOWLEDGE

1. What is the most severe form of asthma?

2. Which category of asthma often occurs in children and may be outgrown?

3. What are some allergens that are found within a dental operatory?

SYMPTOMS

An asthma attack may occur suddenly without any warning or slowly over an extended period of time. The first step when dealing with an asthmatic patient in an emergency situation is to distinguish between asthma and an airway obstruction. If there is confusion, listen to the sounds the patient is making. With airway obstruction, stridor—a constant-pitch musical sound—may be heard during inspirations. With asthma, a wheezing sound heard during expirations is characteristic. In addition, an easy way to determine that the patient is suffering from an asthma attack is to read the health history. If the patient exhibiting signs and symptoms has indicated a history of asthma, the attack should be treated as asthma.

During an asthma attack, the bronchioles become narrowed due to contractions of the smooth muscles, and there is an overproduction of mucus. As a result, the air passages are restricted, breathing becomes difficult, and the patient seems to be struggling for air.

With asthma, exhaling is the most difficult part of breathing, although most of the time the patient feels as if inhaling is the most difficult part.

The patient suffering from an asthma attack may be sweating and coughing, and may appear to be very nervous. The nervousness occurs as a result of the patient's inability to breathe normally. The patient may also complain of a severe tightness in the chest. It is also common for blood pressure and pulse to increase slightly during an attack. However, in some cases, these vital signs may remain close to the baseline readings.

The duration of an asthma attack varies from patient to patient. If left untreated, the attack may continue anywhere from a few minutes to several hours. The patient usually experiences a severe coughing attack and expectorates a large bolus of mucus just before the attack terminates. If the patient is treated immediately with a bronchodilator, the attack usually ends within a few seconds.

Status asthmaticus, as already noted, is the most severe form of asthma. It may begin like any other asthma attack but will not respond to any type of treatment or medication, and the patient therefore experiences one continuous asthma attack. The situation may continue for days. This person is in a life-threatening situation and should be hospitalized immediately.

See Emergency Basics 8-2 for signs and symptoms of asthma.

Emergency Basics 8-2

Asthma Signs and Symptoms

- Coughing
- Sweating
- Tightness in chest
- Difficulty breathing
- Wheezing
- Blood pressure normal or elevated
- Increased heart rate
- Nervousness

TEST YOUR KNOWLEDGE

1. Why is it important to determine the difference between an asthmatic episode and an airway obstruction in an emergency situation?

2. Why does the patient become anxious during an asthma attack?

TREATMENT

Once it has been determined that a patient is suffering from an asthma attack, prompt treatment should be administered as follows:

1. Stop all dental treatment. Be sure to remove all materials and instruments from the patient's mouth. The patient will be breathing forcibly, so make sure there are no cotton rolls or other small items left in the mouth for the patient to inhale.

2. Position the patient. Raise the patient upright; since the patient will be struggling for air, it will be easier for the patient to breathe if seated upright.

bronchodilator
A medication that dilates the bronchioles.

3. Use a **bronchodilator.** The health history will state whether the patient suffers from asthma. Once this information is ascertained, the dental auxiliary should ask the patient whether he or she is carrying a bronchodilator (Figure 8-2a). If so, the patient's bronchodilator should be placed within easy reach in case an attack occurs. If an attack does take place, allow the patient to administer the bronchodilator; patients know what their usual dose involves (Figure 8-2b). The bronchodilator is an aerosol medication that usually includes **epinephrine,** which relaxes the bronchioles and makes it easier for the patient to breathe (Figure 8-3).

epinephrine A vasoconstrictor.

4. Administer oxygen. Administer 4 to 6 liters of oxygen per minute by a full-face mask or nasal cannula, if one is available. Be careful not to frighten the patient when applying the face mask. Asthmatic patients are struggling for air and may get a feeling of suffocation from the oxygen mask. Solve this problem by allowing the patient to hold the mask.

5. If the bronchodilator does not relieve the attack, it may be necessary for the dentist to administer epinephrine or another drug intravenously. The auxiliary should set up the IV according to the dentist's instructions.

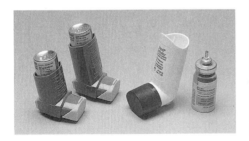
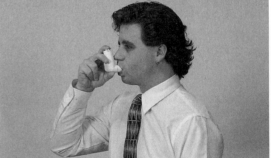

© 2013 Cengage Learning

FIGURE 8-2 (A) Inhalers with bronchodilator medication; (B) patient administering an inhaler during an asthma attack.

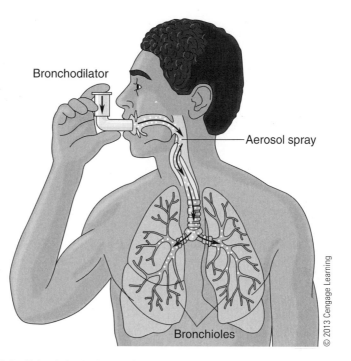

Bronchodilator

Aerosol spray

Bronchioles

© 2013 Cengage Learning

FIGURE 8-3   Epinephrine in the bronchodilator relaxes the bronchioles during an asthma attack.

If these steps are not successful, call for medical assistance. Remember, if all treatment is unsuccessful, the patient may be suffering from status asthmaticus and should be hospitalized as soon as possible.

See Emergency Basics 8-3 for a summary of the treatment for asthma.

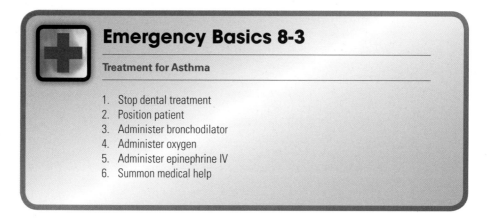

Emergency Basics 8-3

Treatment for Asthma

1. Stop dental treatment
2. Position patient
3. Administer bronchodilator
4. Administer oxygen
5. Administer epinephrine IV
6. Summon medical help

TEST YOUR KNOWLEDGE

1. Where should the patient's bronchodilator be placed during treatment?

2. How should a patient be positioned after it has been determined that the patient is experiencing an asthmatic episode?

SUMMARY

Asthma attacks in the dental office are most often triggered by anxiety. Therefore, it is extremely important to try to keep all patients calm, especially the asthmatic patient. If an asthma attack does occur, try to calm the patient while administering prompt, efficient treatment.

REVIEW QUESTIONS

MULTIPLE CHOICE

1. Which of the following is not a sign or symptom of asthma?
   a. wheezing
   b. tightness in the chest
   c. coughing
   d. stridor

2. A/An _____ may be administered by the patient to relieve asthma.
   a. injection
   b. bronchodilator
   c. IV
   d. tablet

3. What type of asthma is considered the most life-threatening?
   a. status asthmaticus
   b. intrinsic asthma
   c. extrinsic asthma
   d. infectious asthma

4. What type of asthma is usually reported in young children?
   a. extrinsic
   b. infectious
   c. intrinsic
   d. none of the above

5. What type of asthma usually occurs as a result of a bronchial infection?
    a. status asthmaticus
    b. extrinsic asthma
    c. allergic asthma
    d. none of the above

TRUE OR FALSE

_____ 1. An asthma attack may occur suddenly or over a long period of time.

_____ 2. Oxygen should not be administered to the asthmatic patient.

_____ 3. A patient suffering from status asthmaticus should be hospitalized as soon as possible.

_____ 4. Asthma only begins in young children.

_____ 5. Today, all causes of asthma are known.

MEDICAL EMERGENCY!

CASE STUDY 8-1

A 10-year-old male presents with a positive medical history. He has extrinsic asthma. He is in the dental office to have two teeth extracted for orthodontic purposes. The dentist is running behind and the patient has to wait for 20 minutes before he is taken to the operatory. Once there the patient begins to cough, wheeze, and struggle for air. The dentist, aware of the patient's condition, sends the auxiliary to the waiting room to get the bronchodilator from his mother. During this time the dentist stops the treatment and talks calmly to the patient. Once the patient administers his bronchodilator, he recovers completely.

Questions

1. How could keeping the patient waiting in the waiting room add to the chances of the asthma attack occurring?

2.   Where should the patient's bronchodilator have been placed during the treatment?

3.   What was the main cause of the patient's asthma attack?

CASE STUDY 8-2

A 55-year-old female presents in the dental office for a crown preparation with final impressions on tooth number 30. As the auxiliary seats the patient, she asks the patient if there have been any changes in her medical history. The patient states that her physician has given her a bronchodilator. The procedure concludes with no complications and the dentist leaves the treatment room. As the patient is preparing to leave, she begins to cough, and the auxiliary observes that the patient is having difficulty breathing. The auxiliary looks for the patient's bronchodilator.

Questions

1.   What type of asthma attack is the patient most likely experiencing?

2.   What should the auxiliary have done prior to the beginning of treatment?

3.   What was a possible cause of the asthma attack?

4.   What other condition could the patient be experiencing?

CHAPTER 9

Hyperventilation

LEARNING OUTCOMES

Upon completion of this chapter, the student will be able to:

- Define hyperventilation
- Describe the signs and symptoms of hyperventilation
- Explain the causes of hyperventilation
- Explain the treatment of hyperventilation
- Describe the best way to prevent hyperventilation

KEY TERMS

carbon dioxide   diazepam

Hyperventilation is an increase in the rate or depth of breathing that results in a change in the blood chemistry and usually occurs as a result of anxiety. The dental office is an anxious setting for most people, which is why hyperventilation is a very common emergency seen there.

CAUSES

The most common cause of hyperventilation is anxiety. Although not as common, hyperventilation also may be caused by certain physical conditions, emotional upset, or stress.

Hyperventilation is not normally encountered in children. It appears to occur most often in patients who hide their feelings and do not admit their fears of dentistry. In such patients, the anxiety builds up within until they can no longer control it. Children usually cry or scream when frightened, which expresses their fears and prevents hyperventilation from occurring.

PHYSIOLOGY

carbon dioxide
A colorless, odorless gas produced by the oxidation of carbon.

Carbon dioxide in the blood automatically triggers the breathing reflex and stimulates respiration. In this way it helps control the breathing process automatically. A person who begins to hyperventilate increases the depth and rate of respirations much like an athlete who has performed strenuous exercise. By increasing respirations, the person exhales a large amount of carbon dioxide. In the athlete, the exercised muscles release carbon dioxide into the blood, which replenishes the excess given off by the rapid breathing. Because dental patients are motionless, however, they have no way of replenishing the carbon dioxide being exhaled. As a result patients can suffer from a lack of carbon dioxide and have difficulty breathing. When there is a lack of carbon dioxide, the patient must consciously work to inhale and exhale.

Hyperventilation takes place in a cycle. First, the patient becomes very anxious about the dental treatment. This results in the patient beginning to hyperventilate. Next, the patient begins to realize he or she is having difficulty breathing. This then makes the patient more anxious, which worsens the hyperventilation. This cycle will increase in severity unless someone intervenes. It is of utmost importance for members of the dental team to recognize the problem, intervene, and attempt to calm the patient.

TEST YOUR KNOWLEDGE

1. Which group of patients is most unlikely to experience hyperventilation?

2. The patient who hyperventilates is experiencing a lack of what gas?

3. What is the most common cause of hyperventilation?

SIGNS AND SYMPTOMS

A patient first entering the operatory may appear nervous or anxious but usually does not discuss any fear of the dental procedure. The patient begins to breathe deeper and faster. At this point, the patient usually does not realize there has been a change in their breathing pattern. The patient may then complain of a feeling of suffocation and tightness in the chest. As the patient continues to hyperventilate, he or she may experience a feeling of dizziness. If the syndrome is allowed to continue, tingling may develop in the extremities.

Patients experiencing hyperventilation are in respiratory distress, although they will not be cyanotic as in other cases (e.g., an airway obstruction) because they are receiving plenty of oxygen. Their lack of carbon dioxide is the problem in this situation.

See Emergency Basics 9-1 for a summary of the signs and symptoms of hyperventilation.

Emergency Basics 9-1

Signs and Symptoms of Hyperventilation

- Nervousness
- Increase in rate of respirations
- Feeling of suffocation
- Tightness in chest
- Dizziness
- Tingling in extremities

TEST YOUR KNOWLEDGE

1. What are the signs and symptoms of hyperventilation?

2. How do the rate and depth of respiration affect the hyperventilating patient?

TREATMENT

Hyperventilation is an emergency situation that usually can be corrected by performing these steps:

1. Once it has been determined that the patient is hyperventilating, stop all dental treatment. Make sure to remove any objects from the patient's mouth.
2. Place the patient in an upright position. A patient who is having difficulty breathing will be more comfortable sitting upright.

3. Attempt to calm the patient, who will be very agitated and will be breathing rapidly. Explain the condition to the patient. Tell the patient to inhale and hold his or her breath for several seconds before exhaling. This procedure will help increase the level of carbon dioxide.

4. In some cases the patient may be so upset the dental team will not be able to convince the patient to hold his or her breath for even a second. In this situation, increase the level of carbon dioxide by using other techniques. The easiest method is to have the patient breathe into a paper sack. The hyperventilating patient has a sense of suffocation, so be very careful not to startle the patient by placing the bag over the face. Instead, let the patient hold the bag so he or she has a sense of controlling the situation. Once the bag is in place, instruct the patient to breathe in and out of the bag (Figure 9-1). The patient will be inhaling carbon dioxide, and this will help end the episode. Make sure to never use any type of plastic bag.

5. Never administer oxygen to a hyperventilating patient. Remember, this patient already has too much oxygen and too little carbon dioxide.

diazepam A medication used to treat active seizures; also used to treat anxiety, nervousness, and muscle spasms.

6. If the patient is experiencing a severe hyperventilation episode, it may be necessary for the dentist to administer a drug to reduce anxiety. **Diazepam** (Valium) is a commonly prescribed antianxiety drug. If this step is necessary, prepare the prescription and the patient instruction according to the dentist's guidelines.

See Emergency Basics 9-2 for a summary of the treatment for hyperventilation.

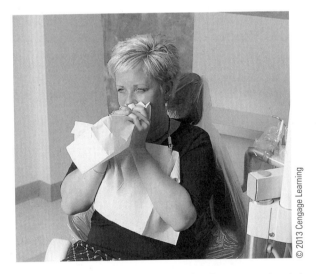

© 2013 Cengage Learning

FIGURE 9-1   A patient who is hyperventilating breathes into a paper bag to increase carbon dioxide into the body.

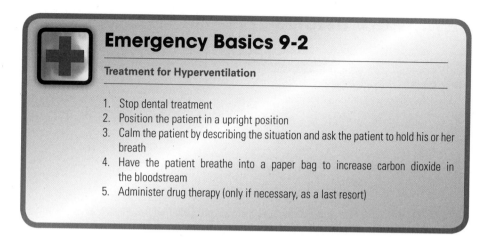

Emergency Basics 9-2

Treatment for Hyperventilation

1. Stop dental treatment
2. Position the patient in a upright position
3. Calm the patient by describing the situation and ask the patient to hold his or her breath
4. Have the patient breathe into a paper bag to increase carbon dioxide in the bloodstream
5. Administer drug therapy (only if necessary, as a last resort)

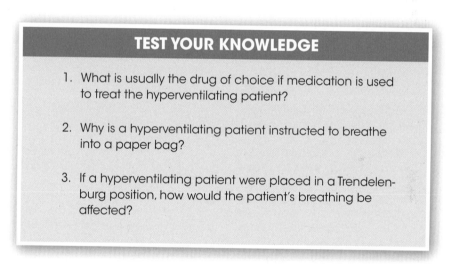

TEST YOUR KNOWLEDGE

1. What is usually the drug of choice if medication is used to treat the hyperventilating patient?

2. Why is a hyperventilating patient instructed to breathe into a paper bag?

3. If a hyperventilating patient were placed in a Trendelenburg position, how would the patient's breathing be affected?

SUMMARY

Hyperventilation in the dental office usually occurs as a result of anxiety. After an episode, it is very important for the dental team to determine what caused the patient's fears of dentistry. Once this has been established, it will be easier for the team to take steps to alleviate the fears and, it is hoped, to prevent another hyperventilation episode.

REVIEW QUESTIONS

MULTIPLE CHOICE

1. Which of the following groups is least likely to experience hyperventilation?
   a. young adults
   b. children
   c. elderly
   d. all the above

2. The patient who hyperventilates is suffering from a lack of
   a. carbon dioxide.
   b. oxygen.
   c. nitrogen.
   d. hydrogen.

3. The most common cause of hyperventilation is
   a. overexertion.
   b. high blood pressure.
   c. lack of oxygen.
   d. none of the above

4. Which of the following is a sign or symptom of hyperventilation?
   a. nervousness
   b. rapid breathing
   c. feeling of suffocation
   d. all the above

5. What is usually the drug of choice if medication is used to treat the hyperventilating patient?
   a. diazepam
   b. Dilantin
   c. epinephrine
   d. none of the above

TRUE OR FALSE

_____   1. Hyperventilation is one of the most uncommon emergencies experienced in the dental office.

_____   2. Hyperventilation usually can be relieved by having the patient breathe into a plastic bag.

_____   3. The rate and depth of respirations increase dramatically in the hyperventilating patient.

_____   4. Hyperventilation usually occurs as a result of a lack of carbon dioxide.

_____   5. The hyperventilating dental patient should be placed in the supine position.

MEDICAL EMERGENCY!

CASE STUDY 9-1

A 35-year-old female patient presents with a negative medical history. She has come to the office to have an amalgam placed in tooth number 20. Once seated in the dental chair, the patient begins to talk rapidly and clutches the arms of the chair. She admits no fear of the dental procedure but appears to be very nervous and then begins to breathe rapidly and complains of tightness in the chest and a feeling of suffocation. She is hyperventilating.

Questions

1. Describe, in order, the type of treatment that should be given to this patient.

2. How could the dental auxiliary prevent this situation from occurring on the patient's next visit?

3.   Why should oxygen not be administered in this situation?

CASE STUDY 9-2

A 25-year-old female presents for routine dental treatment. This appointment is her second visit. On the first visit, she was very anxious, but tolerated the procedures well. At this appointment, the patient is kept waiting in the operatory for a longer period of time due to the duration of another patient's treatment. As the dentist prepares to administer the local anesthesia, the auxiliary notes that the patient is beginning to breathe rapidly and deeply.

Questions

1.   What condition is the patient most likely experiencing?

2.   What is the treatment for this condition?

3.   What could the auxiliary have done to prevent this episode?

CHAPTER 10

Airway Obstruction

LEARNING OUTCOMES

Upon completion of this chapter, the student will be able to:
- Explain several causes of airway obstruction in the dental office
- Explain several ways to prevent airway obstruction in the dental office
- Identify the anatomy of the airway
- Explain the differences between the various types of airway obstructions
- Define the Heimlich maneuver
- Demonstrate the Heimlich maneuver
- Demonstrate manual thrusts
- Demonstrate chest thrusts
- Demonstrate finger sweeps
- Explain the use of the Heimlich on infants
- Explain the use of the Heimlich on children
- Explain the use of the Heimlich on pregnant patients
- Explain the use of the Heimlich on obese patients
- Explain the use of the cricothyrotomy
- Demonstrate how to perform the Heimlich on oneself

KEY TERMS

abdominal thrusts	aspirate	dental dam	trachea
asphyxiation	cyanosis	Heimlich maneuver	tracheotomy

Every aspect of the human body depends on the availability of adequate oxygen to function properly. Depriving the body of oxygen for even a few minutes can lead to irreversible brain damage and ultimately to death. It is therefore of utmost importance to recognize and treat airway obstruction both quickly and correctly. Airway obstruction is not selective; young and old alike can be victims.

DENTAL HAZARDS

aspirate To breathe in forcefully causing an object to become lodged in the airway.

The dental office is a perfect setting for an airway obstruction to occur. The development of sit-down dentistry, which places the patient in the reclining position, has increased the incidence of dental patients **aspirating** objects into the airway. Practically every aspect of dentistry requires that some object be placed into or taken out of the patient's mouth. These objects, when coated with saliva or blood, can easily slip out of the dentist's or auxiliary's hands and cause an obstruction in the patient. Some items that may be aspirated and produce obstructions (see Emergency Basics 10-1) include tooth fragments or whole teeth, amalgam, prosthetic devices, crowns, impression materials, gauze, and cotton rolls.

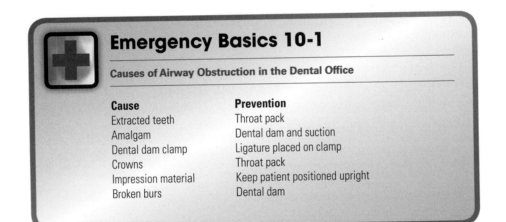

Emergency Basics 10-1

Causes of Airway Obstruction in the Dental Office

Cause	Prevention
Extracted teeth	Throat pack
Amalgam	Dental dam and suction
Dental dam clamp	Ligature placed on clamp
Crowns	Throat pack
Impression material	Keep patient positioned upright
Broken burs	Dental dam

dental dam A thin sheet of latex or nonlatex rubber for isolating one or more teeth during a dental procedure.

The use of certain protective devices such as the **dental dam** or throat packs helps prevent a number of possible airway obstructions. However, some methods of treatment make it impossible to use these devices; in these cases extra precautions must be taken. The auxiliary should be very assertive with the high-volume evacuator and have the cotton pliers available to retrieve any dropped object.

If an object is dropped, it is extremely important to remain calm to keep the patient from overreacting. Most of the time the patient's gag reflex will allow the patient to cough the object back into the mouth where it can be removed.

ANATOMY OF THE AIRWAY

trachea The air passage that descends from the larynx and branches into the right and left bronchi; also known as the *windpipe*.

Most airway obstructions dental personnel encounter occur in the upper airway. To know what occurs during an obstruction, it is important to understand the anatomy of the upper airway. Figure 10-1 is an illustrated view of upper airway anatomy. The mouth and nose empty into a common passage called the pharynx, or throat. At the pharynx two passages extend downward. The first passage is the **trachea.** The trachea is the largest passage, located in the front of the throat, and carries air from the pharynx into the lungs. The second passage is the esophagus, located behind the trachea, which carries solids and liquids from the mouth to the stomach.

When food is swallowed, it is kept out of the trachea by the epiglottis, a flap that covers the opening of the trachea whenever food approaches. In some cases food or other objects get past the epiglottis and pass into the trachea. The majority of the time the patient coughs and the object is removed. However, in some instances the object becomes lodged in the trachea, and an airway obstruction occurs. The upper-airway anatomy is completed by the larynx, or voice box. (The lower airway consists of the bronchi, alveoli, and lungs.)

TYPES OF AIRWAY OBSTRUCTIONS

Airway obstructions can result from a number of situations such as trauma, foreign objects, secretions, burns, or tumors. No matter what the cause, several different types of airway obstructions may occur.

A *partial airway obstruction* occurs when the airway is not completely blocked. In this situation some air gets through to the lungs. A partial obstruction can be one with adequate air exchange or one with inadequate air exchange. A patient experiencing a partial obstruction with adequate air exchange will cough forcibly. This person is able to talk and may try to explain that the object "went down the wrong way." Such a person is usually not in serious trouble.

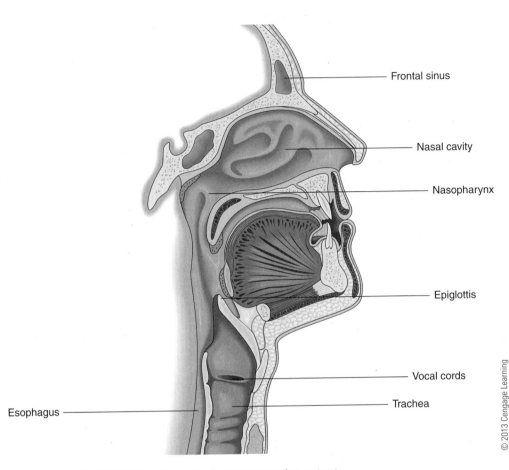

Frontal sinus

Nasal cavity

Nasopharynx

Epiglottis

Vocal cords

Trachea

Esophagus

© 2013 Cengage Learning

FIGURE 10-1   Structures of the upper respiratory tract.

The patient experiencing a *partial obstruction with inadequate air exchange* is certainly in danger. This person will not cough, although a crowing sound will be made that is a result of the air passing over the lodged object. As the episode progresses, the person may show signs of cyanosis around the mouth because of the lack of oxygen. The main problem with this situation is that it can easily become a complete airway obstruction. This patient may not be receiving enough oxygen to sustain life and may lose consciousness, suffer brain damage, or die.

The *complete airway obstruction* is the most life threatening. The individual suffering from this condition is not able to make any noise but may exhibit the universal distress signal, clutching the throat with the hands (Figure 10-2). The person usually panics immediately and may resist treatment. If the obstruction is not removed, the patient loses consciousness quickly. If the oxygen is lacking for about four to six minutes, irreversible brain damage can occur, and ultimately, if the object is not removed, the patient will die.

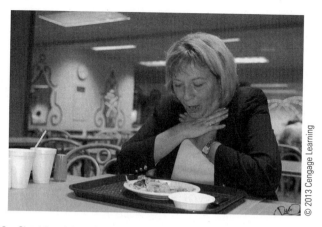

FIGURE 10-2   Clutching the neck with both hands is the universal sign of airway obstruction.

TEST YOUR KNOWLEDGE

1. In which type of airway obstruction can the patient talk and explain the condition?

2. Which type of airway obstruction is the most life threatening?

THE HEIMLICH MANEUVER

Heimlich maneuver
Technique used to remove an object that is lodged in the airway.

Throughout history people have had various remedies for choking; in most cases the treatments were unsuccessful. Dr. Heimlich developed a technique for relieving airway obstructions that has become known as the **Heimlich maneuver** and consists of a series of manual thrusts. The Heimlich maneuver makes use of the air that remains in the victim's lungs. The pressure placed on the abdomen during manual thrusts causes an elevation of the diaphragm, which increases pressure on the lungs and causes an explosive force of air to be released and hopefully to clear the trachea. Since the invention of the Heimlich maneuver, there has been a great deal of controversy over its use. Injuries such as fractured ribs have resulted from the maneuver being performed incorrectly. However, the Heimlich maneuver has been found to be successful unless the object cannot be removed, the maneuver is done incorrectly, or too much time elapsed before the technique was started.

Classifications of Airway Obstructions

The different degrees of airway obstruction outlined earlier require different techniques to treat them.

Partial Obstruction with Adequate Air Exchange This patient coughs forcibly. The only treatment that should be necessary is encouragement to cough. Most of the time, the object is expelled.

Partial Obstruction with Inadequate Air Exchange This patient is in a potentially life-threatening situation, since the obstruction is so great as to prevent the patient from receiving adequate oxygen. This patient should be treated as if suffering from a complete airway obstruction.

cyanosis Bluish skin color that results from decreased oxygen.

asphyxiation Death caused by lack of oxygen.

abdominal thrusts Technique used as part of the Heimlich maneuver, which uses abdominal thrusts to try to dislodge an object.

Complete Airway Obstruction A person suffering from a complete airway obstruction cannot breathe, cannot make any sound, becomes extremely pale and **cyanotic**, and may die from **asphyxiation** in approximately four to six minutes. It is of utmost importance that this condition be diagnosed and treated immediately. In this situation, the best treatment the auxiliary can provide is the Heimlich maneuver plus additional steps. The maneuver consists of: (1) manual thrusts, and (2) finger sweeps (unconscious patient only).

Technique

Manual thrusts may be administered as **abdominal thrusts** or chest thrusts. Both techniques are successful; the patient and the circumstances determine which technique should be used. Chest thrusts are used most often on the pregnant patient or the patient who is extremely obese. Abdominal thrusts may be performed on any other patient.

Abdominal Thrust

- *Conscious Patient*

    1. Stand behind the patient.
    2. Wrap your arms around the patient.
    3. Make a fist with one of your hands.
    4. Place the thumb of the fist against the patient's abdomen halfway between the navel and the rib cage.
    5. Cover the fist with your other hand.
    6. Push the fist quickly four times into the abdomen with an inward and upward motion (see Figures 10-3 and 10-4).

- *Unconscious Patient*

    1. Place the patient in a supine position.
    2. Straddle the patient, facing toward the patient's head. If the patient is small you may stand or kneel alongside.
    3. Place the heel of one hand on the patient's abdomen.
    4. Place the other hand on top of the first hand and interlock the fingers.
    5. Push the heel of the hand rapidly inward and upward four times into the abdomen.

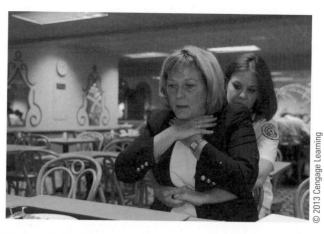

FIGURE 10-3   Stand behind the patient and wrap your arms around the patient's waist.

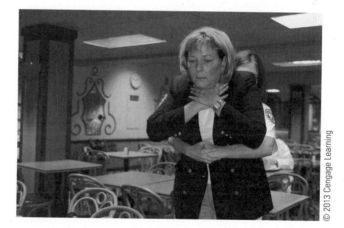

FIGURE 10-4   Place your fist midway between the navel and the rib cage; use an inward and upward motion to dislodge the obstruction.

Chest Thrust

- *Conscious Patient*
    1. Stand behind the patient.
    2. Wrap your arms around the patient.
    3. Make a fist with one hand.
    4. Place the thumb of the fist against the patient's lower sternum. When administering chest thrusts, it is important not to place the hands over the xiphoid process, which could break and cause a laceration of the liver.
    5. Place the other hand over the fist.
    6. Administer four quick thrusts.

- *Unconscious Patient*
  1. Place the patient in the supine position.
  2. Position yourself either beside or straddling the patient.
  3. Place the heel of one hand on the patient's lower sternum. Make sure not to place the hand on the xiphoid process.
  4. Place the other hand on top of the first and interlock the fingers.
  5. Administer four quick downward chest thrusts.

Finger Sweeps   Finger sweeps consist of wiping the patient's oral cavity with the fingers to discover if the obstruction can be reached with your fingers. The procedure is performed only on the unconscious patient. Finger sweeps can be very effective, although they must be used with caution. Care must be taken not to force the object farther down the throat and create a more complete obstruction. Objects should be removed with the fingers only if they are well into the oral cavity and can be easily reached with the fingers.

1. Open the patient's mouth.
2. Use the index and middle fingers.
3. Place the fingers at the corner of the mouth and, using a hooking motion, sweep across the inside of the mouth to the other side.
4. Perform two finger sweeps (see Figure 10-5).

Order of Procedure: Complete Obstruction

- *Conscious Patient*
  1. Stand behind the patient.
  2. Administer four manual thrusts.
  3. Repeat until the object is removed or the patient loses consciousness.

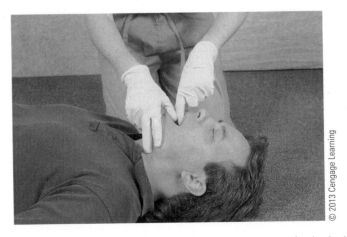

© 2013 Cengage Learning

FIGURE 10-5   Use a sweeping motion with two fingers to remove any foreign body from the patient's mouth.

- ***Unconscious Patient***

  1. Place the patient in the supine position.
  2. Open the airway.
  3. Attempt to ventilate the patient using the mouth-to-mouth technique.
  4. If you are unable to get air into the patient's lungs, reopen the airway and attempt to ventilate again.
  5. Administer four manual thrusts.
  6. Make two finger sweeps.
  7. Repeat the sequence until the object is removed or surgical intervention is performed by trained personnel.

  Note: It is important to continue the Heimlich maneuver even when the patient loses consciousness because the muscles that were constricting and holding the object in place while the patient was conscious may relax during unconsciousness and allow the object to be removed.

  See Emergency Basics 10-2 for a summary of the treatment for airway obstruction.

Emergency Basics 10-2

Summary of Treatment for Airway Obstruction

Partial obstruction—adequate air exchange

1. Encourage the patient to cough as if the patient is experiencing a complete obstruction.

Partial obstruction—inadequate air exchange

1. Treat the condition as if the patient is suffering from a complete obstruction.

Complete airway obstruction

Conscious

1. Four manual thrusts
2. Repeat sequence until object is dislodged or patient loses consciousness

Unconscious

1. Open airway
2. Attempt to ventilate
3. If unable, reposition airway
4. Attempt to ventilate
5. Four manual thrusts
6. Two finger sweeps
7. Repeat sequence

TEST YOUR KNOWLEDGE

1. How does the Heimlich maneuver differ with an unconscious patient?

2. What does the rescuer need to consider when performing finger sweeps on an unconscious patient?

HEIMLICH MANEUVER ON INFANTS AND CHILDREN

Choking is the leading cause of death in infants under one year of age. When administering the Heimlich maneuver on an infant, whether in the dental office or elsewhere, several modifications in technique must be performed. The infant suffering from a complete airway obstruction does not make any sound, turns pale and cyanotic, and collapses due to asphyxiation.

Treatment

- *Conscious Infant*
    1. Place the infant supine on your lap or on a firm surface, depending on your own size.
    2. Place the tips of your index and middle fingers halfway between the infant's navel and rib cage.
    3. Press inward and upward into the abdomen with four quick movements.
    4. If the object is not removed after the four manual thrusts, turn the infant onto its stomach with the head lower than the feet and apply four back blows between the shoulder blades (Figure 10-6).
    5. Repeat the sequence until the infant recovers or loses consciousness.

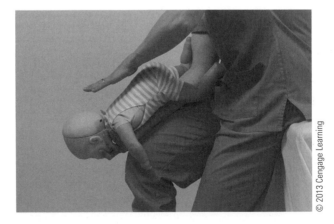

© 2013 Cengage Learning

FIGURE 10-6 Place the infant in a prone position if Steps 1–3 are not successful. Deliver four back blows between the infant's shoulder blades.

- *Unconscious Infant*
  1. Place the infant supine on your lap or on a hard surface, depending on your own size.
  2. Open the airway.
  3. Attempt to ventilate.
  4. If no response, reopen the airway.
  5. Attempt to ventilate.
  6. Place the tips of your index and middle fingers halfway between the infant's navel and rib cage.
  7. Press inward and upward into the abdomen with four quick movements.
  8. Turn the infant onto the stomach with the head lower than the feet and apply four back blows between the shoulder blades.
  9. Using the index finger, perform two finger sweeps if the object is visible in the infant's mouth.
  10. Repeat the sequence until the infant recovers or surgical intervention is performed by trained personnel.

On a child (one through eight years of age), the Heimlich maneuver may be performed the same as on an adult, although it is necessary to reduce the force of all actions. Regardless of where choking occurs, whether in or out of the dental office, the child or infant should be checked by a physician after he or she has recovered to make sure no additional damage has occurred.

Oral Piercing

Body piercing has become a more prevalent form of body art in today's society. Oral piercing, which may involve the tongue, lips, uvula, or a combination of sites, has been implicated in several adverse oral conditions, including:
- gingival injury or recession
- damage to teeth or restorations
- interference with speech or chewing and swallowing
- scar tissue formation
- prolonged bleeding
- severe infection

An emergency related to oral piercing may present in the form of an airway obstruction. The jewelry can become dislodged and move into the airway. When dental personnel are providing treatment for a patient with some form of oral piercing, they should take precautions to avoid dislodging the jewelry.

Because of the potential for various related complications, the American Dental Association opposes the practice of oral piercing.

PATIENTS WITH SPECIAL REQUIREMENTS

Some patients other than infants and children can present problems that require adjustments in the way the Heimlich maneuver is performed.

The first case is the pregnant patient. Not only do you not want to take the chance of damaging the unborn child by applying abdominal thrusts, but the size of the patient sometimes makes it physically impossible to perform the maneuver. Whenever a pregnant patient is suffering from an airway obstruction, the best method of treatment is to perform the Heimlich maneuver exactly as previously stated, except to employ chest thrusts in place of abdominal thrusts. This is the only major adjustment that should be necessary on the pregnant patient. Remember, however, that when the mother is deprived of oxygen, the baby is also deprived. All steps should be taken as quickly as possible to restore oxygen to this patient.

Extremely obese patients also may present specific problems. The size of the patient may prevent manual thrusts while standing behind the patient if you cannot wrap your arms completely around the body. In such cases, all manual thrusts must be performed from the front. To make these steps easier to perform, it is best to have the patient either lying down or seated.

Special circumstances require special actions. The important thing to remember is that a patient can survive for only a very short period of time without oxygen, and the main goal is to do whatever is necessary to clear the obstruction and get oxygen to the patient.

CRICOTHYROTOMY

No matter how well the Heimlich maneuver is performed, in some situations it is not successful. If such a situation arises, it may be necessary to use surgical intervention. Any type of surgical airway intervention, however, should only be done by someone qualified in its use, and only as a last resort.

tracheotomy
Incision made through the skin into the trachea to relieve an airway obstruction.

Formerly the method of choice was a **tracheotomy,** but the area where it must be performed is very close to several large sources of blood and nerve supplies, and therefore this technique can easily cause severe problems even when performed in the best of circumstances, to say nothing of an emergency situation. As a result, the cricothyrotomy has replaced the tracheotomy as the treatment of choice when an emergency airway must be provided. A cricothyrotomy is performed as follows:

1. Locate the cricothyroid membrane by placing the finger on the Adam's apple and sliding downward toward the feet until you feel a slight indented area. This is the cricothyroid membrane.
2. Using a sharp object, preferably a scalpel, make an incision in this area, and then widen the incision. There will be little bleeding because there are no major blood vessels in this area.
3. The opening must be maintained. Place an item such as a suction tip or your finger into the incision to keep the airway open. If necessary, artificial respiration may be administered through this temporary air space.

A modification of this technique is use of the cricothyrotomy needle. Practically every emergency kit contains such an item. The needle has a very large diameter, which permits air to pass through. The method detailed above is used with one exception: instead of making an incision, the needle is inserted into the cricothyroid membrane.

PERFORMING THE HEIMLICH ON YOURSELF

Manual thrusts may be performed on yourself if you are choking and no help is available.

1. Place your hands in the position described for abdominal thrusts, and press.
2. Place yourself against the banister of a stairway, corner of a sink, or arm of a chair and press quickly against it. These techniques are by no means as effective as the full Heimlich maneuver but may prove effective when no other means of help is available.

SUMMARY

An airway obstruction can occur at any time to any patient. Brain damage or death can occur very quickly as a result of an airway obstruction. It is therefore of utmost importance that the dental auxiliary quickly recognize and effectively treat the condition.

REVIEW QUESTIONS

MULTIPLE CHOICE

1. The trachea is commonly known as the
   a. voice box.
   b. throat.
   c. windpipe.
   d. none of the above

2. Which of the following is true concerning a partial obstruction with inadequate air exchange?
   (1) patient may exhibit a crowing sound
   (2) should be treated as a complete obstruction
   (3) is not a serious condition
   (4) patient may be cyanotic
   a. 1, 2, 3, 4
   b. 1, 2, 3
   c. 2, 3, 4
   d. 1, 2, 4

3. What should be the treatment for a patient suffering from a partial obstruction with adequate air exchange?
   a. encourage coughing
   b. administer two finger sweeps
   c. use the full Heimlich
   d. use manual thrusts only

4. Which of the following is true concerning finger sweeps?
   a. administer finger sweeps only to infants
   b. finger sweeps are performed only on unconscious victims
   c. use two fingers to perform finger sweeps
   d. b and c

5. It would be best to use chest thrusts on the
   a. pregnant patient.
   b. tall patient.
   c. unconscious patient.
   d. all the above

6. The universal distress signal to indicate an airway obstruction is
   a. placing the palm of the hand over the mouth.
   b. clutching the throat with both hands.
   c. covering the eyes with the palms of both hands.
   d. none of the above

7. Which of the following techniques is performed only on the unconscious patient?
   (1) chest thrusts
   (2) finger sweeps
   (3) artificial respirations
   (4) manual thrusts
   a. 1, 2
   b. 2, 3, 4
   c. 2, 3
   d. 3, 4

8. The tips of the index and middle fingers are used to administer manual thrusts on
   a. elderly patients.
   b. obese patients.
   c. pregnant patients.
   d. infants.

9. What is the most accepted surgical technique for relieving an airway obstruction?
   a. cricothyrotomy
   b. tracheotomy
   c. laryngectomy
   d. none of the above

10. Abdominal thrusts should be administered
    a. over the diaphragm.
    b. over the lower sternum.
    c. between the sternum and diaphragm.
    d. between the navel and rib cage.

TRUE OR FALSE

_____   1. Brain damage can occur as a result of a lack of oxygen in as little as four to six minutes.

_____   2. The use of the rubber dam may help prevent some airway obstructions.

_____   3. It is best to perform manual thrusts while standing in front of the patient.

_____   4. The Heimlich maneuver is usually not successful when performed on infants and children.

_____   5. The Heimlich maneuver should be stopped once a patient loses consciousness.

_____   6. The universal distress signal consists of the victim's clutching the throat with the hands.

_____   7. The unconscious patient should be placed in the upright position before administering the Heimlich.

_____   8. Chest thrusts are best performed on obese and pregnant patients.

_____   9. Finger sweeps performed incorrectly can force the foreign object back into the victim's throat.

_____ 10. You should attempt to ventilate both a conscious and an unconscious patient.

MEDICAL EMERGENCY!

CASE STUDY 10-1

A 16-year-old male presents in the dental office with a negative medical history. He has come to the dental office to have a crown cemented on number 30. During the try-in the crown slips from the dentist's hand and enters the patient's throat. The patient begins to gasp and make a crowing sound. The dental team gets the patient out of the chair and begins to perform the Heimlich. After two sequences, the object is expelled and the patient recovers.

Questions

1.   What type of obstruction is the patient experiencing?

2.   What could have been done to prevent this situation from occurring?

3.   Explain the steps, in the correct order, of the procedure that would be performed on this patient.

CASE STUDY 10-2

A 32-year-old female presents in the dental office with a positive medical history. She is in her second trimester and is six months pregnant. The patient is scheduled to have impressions made for a whitening tray. The dental auxiliary places the patient in a supine position and inserts the upper impression tray. The patient begins choking and experiencing airway obstruction with inadequate air exchange.

Questions

1.   How could this emergency have been prevented?

2.   What modifications of the Heimlich maneuver should be performed with this patient?

3.   What additional considerations should be taken with this patient due to her medical history?

SECTION FOUR

Cardiovascular Emergencies

This section deals with medical conditions and emergencies that involve the cardiovascular system.

CHAPTER 11

Angina Pectoris and Myocardial Infarction

LEARNING OUTCOMES

Upon completion of this chapter, the student will be able to:

- Name the major parts of the heart
- Explain how atherosclerosis affects the coronary arteries
- Describe the progression of coronary artery disease
- Define angina pectoris
- Explain the difference between stable and unstable angina
- List three precipitating factors of angina
- Describe the signs and symptoms of angina
- Explain how the dentist may diagnose angina
- Describe the treatment for angina
- List two side effects of nitroglycerin
- Define myocardial infarction
- Describe the signs and symptoms of myocardial infarction
- Describe the treatment for myocardial infarction
- Describe the three differences between angina and myocardial infarction
- Explain how stress is a precipitating factor of angina
- Explain what the dental team can do to prevent angina or myocardial infarction from occurring in the dental office

KEY TERMS

amyl nitrite	atrioventricular valves	myocardial infarction	semilunar valves
angina pectoris	coronary artery disease	myocardium	vasodilator
aorta	endocardium	nitroglycerin	ventricles
arteriosclerosis	epicardium	orthostatic hypotension	
atherosclerosis	epigastrium	pericardium	
atria	lumen	pulmonary artery	

Today the mere mention of heart attack, heart disease, or cardiovascular disease strikes fear into most people. This fear is not entirely unjustified, since cardiovascular disease is the major cause of death in the United States today. Heart disease may present itself in several ways, but this chapter is limited to two types of heart disease that may present emergency situations in the dental office: angina pectoris and acute myocardial infarction.

ANATOMY OF THE HEART

pericardium
Sac that encloses the heart.

epicardium
Inner layer of the pericardium.

myocardium
Middle layer of the heart wall.

endocardium
Lining of the inner heart surface.

atria Upper chambers of the heart.

ventricles Lower chambers of the heart.

To understand how certain diseases or conditions affect the heart, it is important to understand some of the basic anatomy of the heart.

Several structures combine to make up the four-chambered, hollow, muscular organ known as the heart. First, the **pericardium** is the wall, or sac, that encloses the heart. This wall is made up of three layers: the external layer, called the **epicardium**; the middle layer, called the **myocardium**; and the inner layer, called the **endocardium** (see Figure 11-1). Each layer has special characteristics or responsibilities. First, coronary vessels must pass through the epicardium before entering the myocardium. Second, the myocardium consists of muscle fibers that give the heart the ability to contract. Third, the endocardium lines the cavities of the heart, covers the valves, and, to some extent, lines the large blood vessels.

The heart consists of four chambers. The upper chambers are called the **atria** and are separated into right and left sides by the interatrial septum. The lower chambers are called the **ventricles** and are divided into right and left sides by the interventricular septum. Refer to Figure 11-2 for anatomy of the human heart.

The right atrium receives blood from all tissues except the lungs. This blood is then pumped to the right ventricle, from which the **pulmonary artery** exits and carries blood to the lungs. The left atrium receives oxygenated blood from the lungs by way of the

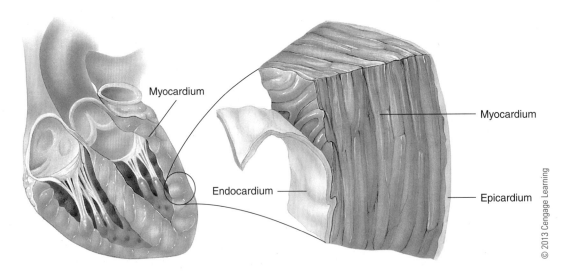

Myocardium

Myocardium

Endocardium

Epicardium

© 2013 Cengage Learning

FIGURE 11-1 Types of tissues that make up the heart muscle: myocardium and epicardium.

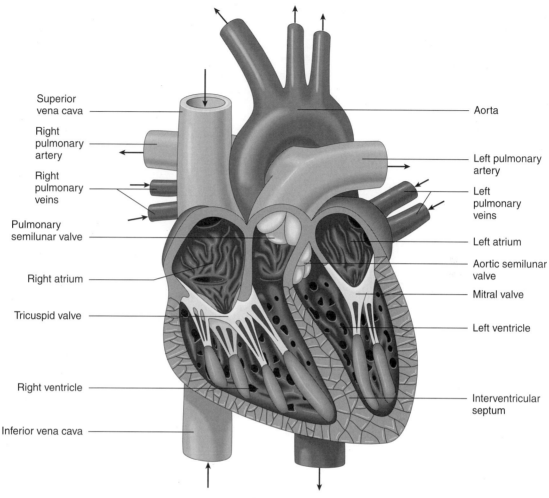

FIGURE 11-2   Anatomy of the human heart.

pulmonary artery
Artery that runs
from the right
ventricle to the
lungs.

aorta Main
artery of the
human body.

**atrioventricular
valve** A valve in
the heart through
which blood flows
from the atria to
the ventricles.

pulmonary veins. The left ventricle is connected to the **aorta,** which pumps blood to all parts of the body except the lungs.

Contained within the heart's chambers are two kinds of valves: the **atrioventricular valves,** which consist of the tricuspid and mitral valves, and the **semilunar valves,** which consist of the pulmonary and aortic valves. The atrioventricular valves separate the atria from the ventricles. The right atrium and ventricle are separated by the tricuspid valve, and the left atrium and ventricle are separated by the mitral valve. The valves allow blood to be pumped from the atria to the ventricles when the atria contract and then prevent blood from reversing when the ventricles contract.

The semilunar valves work similarly, although their location is different. The pulmonary valve is located between the right ventricle and the pulmonary artery, and the aortic valve is located between the left ventricle and the aorta.

semilunar valves
Valves with half-moon-shaped cusps, for example, the aortic valve and the pulmonary valve.

The heart is best known as the organ that provides blood to the rest of the body, but, in order to survive, the heart muscle itself must receive an adequate supply of oxygenated blood. The myocardium is supplied with blood by the first branches of the aorta, the right and left coronary arteries. The left coronary artery branches to supply blood to the left and right ventricles and left atrium. The right coronary artery branches and supplies blood to the left and right ventricles and the right atrium.

CORONARY ARTERY DISEASE

arteriosclerosis
Thickening of the artery walls that results in loss of elasticity.

atherosclerosis
Form of arteriosclerosis that affects the coronary arteries and causes coronary artery disease.

coronary artery disease A condition in which the walls of the coronary arteries become thick and hard.

lumen The cavity of a tubular organ such as a blood vessel.

Both physical and emotional stress can cause the heart to work harder and therefore require more oxygen. In a healthy heart this is not a problem, because the vessels dilate and the heart receives more oxygenated blood on call. However, when the heart is diseased, this dilation does not take place.

A common disease that causes this problem is **arteriosclerosis,** more commonly called hardening of the arteries, in which the artery walls become thickened and inelastic (also discussed in Chapter 7). **Atherosclerosis** is the form of arteriosclerosis that affects the coronary arteries and causes **coronary artery disease.** With this condition, the walls of the coronary arteries become thick and hard. The process is usually gradual and may take years to develop. The process begins with small amounts of fatty deposits or plaques in the arteries that with time increase in size and cause a narrowing of the opening or **lumen** of the arteries. Calcification follows, and eventually the diameter of the artery becomes dangerously small.

The degree of this narrowing and the severity of the coronary artery disease determine the adverse effects the patient experiences. For example, with a narrowing of the arteries, the patient may experience angina pectoris. However, if the artery is extremely narrow or perhaps even occluded, myocardial infarction may occur. Coronary artery disease can progress. A patient may experience angina for a period of time and then, as the disease increases in severity, experience a myocardial infarction.

TEST YOUR KNOWLEDGE

1. What layer of the heart enables the heart to contract?

2. What is the difference between arteriosclerosis and atherosclerosis?

3. How does the progression of fatty deposits affect the disease process?

ANGINA PECTORIS

angina pectoris
A severe pain in and around the heart caused by an insufficient supply of oxygenated blood to the heart.

Angina pectoris is a Latin phrase that means a "strangling of the chest." Angina is characterized by episodes of pain when the heart experiences oxygen deficiency. This oxygen deficiency may be caused by conditions that result in decreased blood flow to the heart, decreased capacity of the blood to carry oxygen, or increased workload in the heart. A diminishment of the oxygen supply to the heart muscle results in myocardial ischemia or hypoxia. In some cases, angina is the first sign of atherosclerotic disease of the coronary arteries.

Signs and Symptoms

epigastrium
Area of the upper abdomen.

The most common symptom of angina is pain, usually in the substernal area of the chest, although it can be located anywhere in the chest from the **epigastrium** to the base of the neck. That the pain may spread to the jaw and teeth should be of some concern to the dental team. In these situations, it is not unusual for even an edentulous (without teeth) patient to consult a dentist with continuous jaw pain. Some patients may describe the condition as a pressure or tightness in the chest rather than as actual pain.

The duration of the pain associated with angina is just as important as the location. An angina episode usually lasts 3 to 5 minutes if the precipitating factors are removed. If the factors are not removed, the episode may last up to 40 minutes. If the episode continues much longer, the possibility of a myocardial infarction should be considered.

During an episode, the patient usually remains motionless in an attempt to alleviate the pain. In most cases the pain ceases within minutes, and the patient may continue activity. However, if the patient does not stop activity at least for a short period, the pain worsens until it becomes almost unbearable. On the other hand, in a few patients the pain may stop without cessation of the physical activity. This recovery can be possible because the collateral channels may start to function, which decreases myocardial hypoxia. The increase in the oxygen levels that are occurring with alternate pathways will help to reduce the patient's discomfort and pain.

The physical signs in an angina attack usually are not very reliable. Appearance may remain relatively normal, or the patient's skin may appear pale or gray in color and become cold and clammy. The pulse rate and blood pressure may increase slightly before or coincidentally with the onset of an angina attack. The increase in pulse rate and blood

TEST YOUR KNOWLEDGE

1. What will occur as a result of the heart muscle experiencing hypoxia?

2. What is a common first sign of atherosclerotic disease of the coronary arteries?

pressure is the central nervous system's way of trying to increase the oxygen flow to the myocardium. The patient may also experience a feeling of impending doom.

See Emergency Basics 11-1 for a summary of the signs and symptoms of angina.

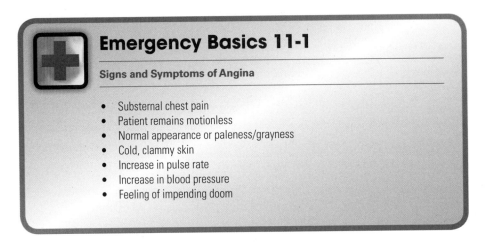

Emergency Basics 11-1

Signs and Symptoms of Angina

- Substernal chest pain
- Patient remains motionless
- Normal appearance or paleness/grayness
- Cold, clammy skin
- Increase in pulse rate
- Increase in blood pressure
- Feeling of impending doom

Classifications of Angina

nitroglycerin
A coronary vasodilator frequently prescribed for the prevention or relief of angina.

Angina pectoris is most often classified as either stable or unstable. Pain from stable angina usually occurs as a result of physical exertion or emotional upset. Stable angina usually does not alter in frequency, duration, or intensity within a 60-day period, whereas unstable angina changes. Unstable angina is unpredictable in regard to cause, with episodes occurring even at rest. Attacks often increase in frequency, severity, and duration. Attacks that were once controlled by **nitroglycerin** may require a higher dosage or become completely immune to its effects. See Emergency Basics 11-2 for a comparison of stable and unstable angina.

Emergency Basics 11-2

Comparison of Stable and Unstable Angina

Stable Angina

1. Pain results from physical or emotional stress
2. No alteration in duration, frequency, or intensity
3. Controlled with nitroglycerin

Unstable Angina

1. Pain may occur even at rest
2. Often increases in duration, frequency, or intensity
3. May require increase in dosage of nitroglycerin, or nitroglycerin may have no effect

Precipitating Factors of Angina Episodes

Classically, angina occurs following physical exertion or emotional stress. Eating or drinking something cold may also trigger an attack. Other activities that may bring on an attack are bathing, dressing, and sex. The amount of stress necessary to cause an attack can vary from time to time, and an angina episode may occur at any time of day or night. A person may experience an attack immediately after going to bed as a result of the effort used to undress or bathe or on waking in the morning after disturbing dreams.

Emotional tension plays a major role as a precipitating factor of angina. In addition, chest discomfort from a stressful situation tends to last longer than that caused by physical exertion because emotions are not as easy to control as physical activity.

See Emergency Basics 11-3 for a summary of precipitating factors of angina episodes.

Emergency Basics 11-3

Precipitating Factors of Angina Episodes

1. Physical exertion
2. Emotional stress
3. Eating or drinking cold foods
4. Dressing
5. Bathing
6. Sexual activity
7. Disturbing dreams

Diagnosis

If the patient experiences chest pain while in the dental office, the dentist must attempt to determine the cause. The first course of action is to recheck the patient's medical history for any notations of angina or other cardiac problems. If the health history is of no help, one solution is to ask the patient certain crucial questions:

1. *What type of discomfort are you experiencing?* It is best not to ask what type of pain the patient is experiencing because some people may not describe the condition as pain. Rather, they may describe the condition as being like a vise clamping down on the chest or like someone standing on the chest. Others may describe the condition as a dull, burning sensation. If the patient describes a sharp or knifelike pain, the condition is probably not angina pectoris.
2. *Describe the location of your discomfort.* Angina pectoris pain is not usually well localized. If the patient can point to one small area where the pain is occurring, the problem is most likely not angina. Most often angina is felt in the substernal area in the middle of the chest. The pain may radiate down either or both arms and may cause a feeling of numbness. The pain may also radiate to the neck or jaw.

3. *How long did your discomfort last?* Angina pain is usually steady, with very little change in intensity, and may last from a minute to several hours. However, the longer the pain lasts, the greater the chances of the patient experiencing a myocardial infarction. Pain that fluctuates or lasts only a few seconds is usually not angina.

4. *What preceded the discomfort?* Angina pain is usually brought on by physical exertion or emotional stress. Exposure to cold weather or eating a large meal may also be a precipitating factor. It is beneficial for the dental team to be aware of the precipitating factors to prevent a recurrence of the attack.

5. *What provided relief from your discomfort?* If relief comes after resting for a few minutes, taking nitroglycerin, or both, the condition is most likely angina. Remember, however, that this is a very tricky situation, since some other serious heart conditions may mimic these symptoms.

Some of these questions may not be appropriate if the patient is experiencing an angina episode, since the symptoms for a myocardial infarction may result in different answers.

Since the basic symptoms of most heart conditions are very similar, the emergency diagnosis may depend on the patient's response to certain treatment. For example, if the patient is treated with nitroglycerin and the pain is not relieved, the condition may be myocardial infarction rather than angina.

TEST YOUR KNOWLEDGE

1. What are characteristics of unstable angina pectoris?

2. What are precipitating factors of angina pectoris?

3. What is the most common symptom of angina pectoris?

Treatment

Once the dentist has diagnosed the patient's condition as angina pectoris, the goal of treatment must be to reduce the demand of the heart muscle for oxygen. This is achieved by these steps:

1. Remain calm. It is vital that the patient have confidence in the ability of the dental team to manage the situation, especially if this is the first time the patient has experienced an angina attack. The dental team should alleviate as much anxiety as possible.

2. Stop all dental treatment. Make sure to remove all items from the patient's mouth. Also make sure to remove from the patient's sight all items that may have been causing concern or anxiety, such as syringes.

3. Position the patient. Place the patient in whatever position is most comfortable.

4. Administer nitroglycerin. Ask patients who have reported a medical history of angina if they have their nitroglycerin with them, and if they do, place the medication within

easy reach. Most emergency kits contain nitroglycerin, but it is best that patients administer their own, since the dosage has been determined to meet their needs. The nitroglycerin should be placed sublingually and allowed to dissolve.

5. Administer oxygen. Since the patient is suffering from a lack of oxygenated blood reaching the heart, administering oxygen makes the patient more comfortable.

6. If the angina is not relieved by the first dose of nitroglycerin, a second dose may be administered.

7. If the treatment described is unsuccessful in relieving the patient's symptoms, the dental team should assume the patient is experiencing myocardial infarction rather than angina and treat accordingly.

amyl nitrite
A vasodilator.

Note: If nitroglycerin is not available, **amyl nitrite** may be administered. However, in some instances unpleasant side effects have been associated with this drug, so administer it only if nitroglycerin is not available. Side effects of amyl nitrite can include spontaneous voiding of the bladder, loss of sphincter control of the large intestine, nausea, vomiting, syncope, hypotension, and an abnormally fast heart rate.

See Emergency Basics 11-4 for a summary of the procedure for treatment of angina.

Emergency Basics 11-4

Treatment of Angina

1. Remain calm
2. Stop dental treatment
3. Position patient
4. Administer nitroglycerin
5. Administer oxygen
6. Administer second dose of nitroglycerin if needed, or amyl nitrite
7. Summon medical assistance if necessary

Nitroglycerin

vasodilator
An agent that causes the dilation of blood vessels.

Nitroglycerin is a coronary **vasodilator** prescribed for the prevention or relief of angina. Its function is to help dilate the coronary arteries to allow more oxygenated blood to reach the heart. Sublingual nitroglycerin has become the accepted drug for the relief of angina episodes because of its rapid action. Nitroglycerin that is administered sublingually can be rapidly absorbed through the highly vascularized mucosa under the tongue. On the average, effects of nitroglycerin are noticeable within 90 seconds after sublingual administration of the correct dose.

Nitroglycerin also can be administered in pill form, as a spray, or through a transdermal patch. The transdermal patch is placed on clean dry skin once a day and is commonly used in the prophylactic treatment of angina (see Figure 11-3). Some patients may use a topical ointment form of nitroglycerin, which they place on the chest before participating in a physical activity they feel may trigger an attack.

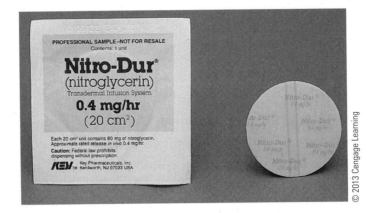

FIGURE 11-3 Transdermal nitroglycerin patch Nitro-Dur® is one way to manage angina pectoris.

Individual sensitivity to nitroglycerin varies, so a physician will determine the correct dose for each individual. For this reason, it is important to allow patients to administer their own nitroglycerin if possible.

Two common side effects are associated with the use of nitroglycerin. First, **orthostatic hypotension** can occur (it may be corrected with dose adjustments). Second, severe headaches may result when nitroglycerin administration is first started. Most clinicians have observed the disappearance of these initial headaches during the continued administration of the nitroglycerin.

Nitroglycerin should improve the patient's condition within about a minute and a half after it is administered. If it is not effective, the nitroglycerin may be old (which is why nitroglycerin should be stored in its original bottle with the cap tightly sealed) or the atherosclerosis may be so severe that the drug is no longer effective and other medication may be needed. Although nitroglycerin alone allows most angina sufferers to lead normal lives, in some cases additional drugs, such as beta blockers, may also be required.

orthostatic hypotension Decrease in blood pressure when a person is raised supine to erect.

TEST YOUR KNOWLEDGE

1. What is the most common medication used to treat angina pectoris?

2. What effect does it have on the coronary arteries that makes it the drug of choice for a patient having an angina attack?

3. What is the treatment for a patient who is experiencing an angina attack?

MYOCARDIAL INFARCTION

myocardial infarction
Circulatory emergency caused by occlusion of at least one of the coronary arteries.

As mentioned earlier, atherosclerosis causes a narrowing of the coronary vessels. When this condition is not severe, angina usually occurs. However, when there is a significant narrowing or a blockage of the coronary arteries, a condition known as **myocardial infarction** may occur. Myocardial infarction is included in the section with angina because in some cases angina attacks may advance to myocardial infarction. On the other hand, myocardial infarction may occur in a patient who has never experienced an angina episode.

Myocardial infarction is a condition that occurs when a portion of the myocardium dies as a result of oxygen starvation caused by the narrowing or complete blockage of the artery that supplies that area with blood (refer to Figure 11-4 for a detailed illustration). The condition may be created by any problem that causes an inadequate supply of oxygenated blood to reach the myocardium, a very common cause being atherosclerosis.

TEST YOUR KNOWLEDGE

1. What is occurring to the heart muscle during a myocardial infarction?

2. Why is the heart muscle experiencing this occurrence?

Signs and Symptoms

The pain associated with myocardial infarction most often occurs when the patient is at rest. When questioned after this type of episode, most patients report that they experienced angina-type pain hours to days prior to the myocardial infarction. The compressing, squeezing pain usually begins in the substernal area and then spreads to other areas. The pain associated with myocardial infarction may vary in degree from severe to almost nonexistent. It may last for 30 minutes or may even continue until analgesic medication is administered. This pain is not relieved by nitroglycerin.

Furthermore, the patient may have cold and clammy skin, vomiting, nausea, dizziness, or hypotension and may exhibit shortness of breath, sweating, weakness, extreme fatigue, anxiety, and a feeling of impending doom. In the final stages, the patient may pass through stupor, coma, and ultimately death.

See Emergency Basics 11-5 for a summary of the signs and symptoms of myocardial infarction.

Treatment

Treatment of myocardial infarction is achieved by these steps:

1. Remain calm. As with any emergency situation, it is important that the patient have confidence in your ability.
2. Stop all dental treatment. Make sure to remove all materials and equipment from in and around the patient's mouth.

Cross-sections through a coronary artery
undergoing progressive atherosclerosis
and arteriosclerosis

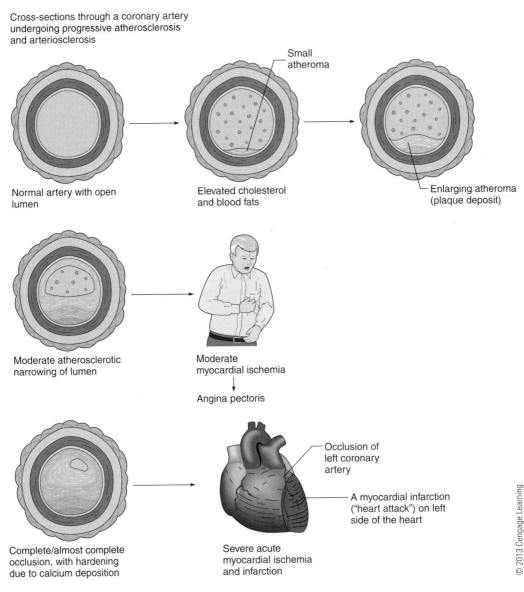

Normal artery with open
lumen

Small
atheroma

Elevated cholesterol
and blood fats

Enlarging atheroma
(plaque deposit)

Moderate atherosclerotic
narrowing of lumen

Moderate
myocardial ischemia

Angina pectoris

Complete/almost complete
occlusion, with hardening
due to calcium deposition

Severe acute
myocardial ischemia
and infarction

Occlusion of
left coronary
artery

A myocardial infarction
("heart attack") on left
side of the heart

© 2013 Cengage Learning

FIGURE 11-4   The progression of coronary heart disease resulting in a myocardial infarction.

3. Administer nitroglycerin. Remember that several heart conditions present with similar symptoms. Administering nitroglycerin aids in diagnosis because nitroglycerin does not relieve the pain of myocardial infarction.

4. Summon medical assistance. A person experiencing a myocardial infarction requires hospital care.

Emergency Basics 11-5

Signs and Symptoms of Myocardial Infarction

- Pain usually occurs at rest
- Compressing, squeezing pain beginning in substernal area and spreading
- Severity of pain varies
- Pain is not relieved by nitroglycerin
- Cold, clammy skin
- Vomiting
- Nausea
- Sweating
- Weakness or extreme fatigue
- Feeling of impending doom

5. Keep the patient as quiet and calm as possible. Some patients suffering myocardial infarction may move about in an effort to get comfortable. However, it is of utmost importance to try to keep the patient from placing any additional stress or strain on the heart.
6. Position the patient. Most myocardial infarction victims are most comfortable in a seated position.
7. Provide oxygen. This helps the patient rest more comfortably.
8. Assist patients in taking their medication if they are under a doctor's care.
9. Be prepared for any complication, including cardiac arrest.
    See Emergency Basics 11-6 for a summary of the procedure for treatment of myocardial infarction.

Emergency Basics 11-6

Treatment of Myocardial Infarction

1. Stop dental treatment
2. Administer nitroglycerin
3. Summon medical assistance if nitroglycerin does not relieve pain
4. Keep patient quiet and calm
5. Position patient
6. Provide oxygen
7. Be prepared to perform CPR

> ### TEST YOUR KNOWLEDGE
>
> 1. What is a key event that will indicate to the dental team that the patient is experiencing more than angina pectoris?
>
> 2. How would the dental auxiliary position the patient if it is suspected that the patient is experiencing a myocardial infarction?

ANGINA AND MYOCARDIAL INFARCTION

Differences

Being aware of the differences between angina and myocardial infarction will help the dental team in determining which one a patient is experiencing. These differences include:

1. The pain associated with myocardial infarction is usually greater in severity and duration than with angina.
2. Myocardial infarction pain occurs in the absence of physical exertion or emotional stress.
3. The patient who is experiencing myocardial infarction continues to move about, trying to find a comfortable position, whereas the angina patient remains motionless.

> ### TEST YOUR KNOWLEDGE
>
> 1. What are the signs and symptoms in a patient who may be experiencing myocardial infarction?
>
> 2. Why does the patient experience extreme pain during a myocardial infarction?

Prevention

The patient experiencing angina, especially the first time, is very frightened and upset. Most associate the chest discomfort with impending death, primarily because most people know someone who has died from a heart problem. This concern increases the need for oxygen going to the heart and therefore has a tendency to worsen the condition. The dental team must work to relieve the fear brought about by this association. This may be accomplished by prompt treatment to relieve the chest discomfort, maintaining control of the situation, and reassuring the patient.

It is always better to try to prevent an angina attack from occurring in the dental office than to have to treat an episode, because an angina attack can lead to myocardial infarction and even to death. Prevention is accomplished by being aware of the patient's medical history and taking steps to alleviate stress from the dental visit.

With all dental patients, it is important to try to make the visit pain-free, but this is especially important with patients who have a history of coronary problems. Pain tends to cause stress, which will aggravate a heart condition and possibly trigger an attack. It may be necessary to limit the length of dental appointments for heart patients, since the stress placed on such patients by long appointments may trigger an attack.

SUMMARY

Heart disease is the leading cause of death in the United States today and is therefore a possible emergency the dental team may have to deal with. Angina is a condition most patients are aware that they have and will note on the health history. In these situations, the dental team should do everything possible to alleviate undue stress, which may trigger an angina episode. It is certainly more beneficial to prevent an angina attack from occurring than to treat it once it happens. Angina, allowed to progress without proper treatment, may escalate to myocardial infarction. At the same time, myocardial infarction can occur without the patient having a history of angina. The dental team should try to prevent as much stress as possible and then be aware of the signs, symptoms, and treatment for a cardiac emergency in case it occurs while a patient is in the dental office.

REVIEW QUESTIONS

MULTIPLE CHOICE

1. The layer of the wall of the heart that gives the heart the ability to contract is the
   a. epicardium.
   b. myocardium.
   c. endocardium.
   d. pericardium.

2. Which of the following is not a characteristic of unstable angina?
   a. episodes may occur at rest
   b. no alteration in frequency
   c. may require higher dose of nitroglycerin
   d. episodes often increase in intensity and duration

3. Which of the following is a precipitating factor of angina?
   a. drinking a cold drink
   b. sexual activity
   c. walking
   d. all the above

4. When treating patients experiencing an angina attack, it is best to give the patients their own nitroglycerin because
    a. the office supply of nitroglycerin should be saved for patients who are not taking nitroglycerin.
    b. you will be assured that the nitroglycerin has not expired.
    c. the dosage will be adjusted for that particular patient.
    d. none of the above

5. If all the normal treatment for angina does not relieve the pain, the dental team should assume that the patient is suffering from
    a. cerebrovascular accident.
    b. cardiac arrest.
    c. respiratory distress.
    d. myocardial infarction.

6. The coronary vasodilator most commonly used to treat angina is
    a. insulin.
    b. nitroglycerin.
    c. bronchodilator.
    d. epinephrine.

7. Which of the following is not a sign or symptom of myocardial infarction?
    a. most often occurs following physical exertion or emotional stress
    b. compressing, squeezing pain in the substernal area
    c. may last in duration for 30 minutes or more
    d. feeling of impending doom

8. When positioning the patient experiencing myocardial infarction, it is best to place the patient in a _____ position.
    a. supine
    b. seated
    c. standing
    d. none of the above

9. The syndrome characterized by episodes of pain when the heart experiences oxygen deficiency is
    a. cardiac arrest.
    b. myocardial infarction.
    c. pulmonary edema.
    d. none of the above

10. Which of the following is a sign or symptom of angina?
    a. substernal chest pain
    b. patient remains motionless
    c. increase in blood pressure
    d. all the above

TRUE OR FALSE

_____ 1. Atherosclerosis is the form of arteriosclerosis that affects the coronary arteries and causes coronary artery disease.

_____ 2. The amount of stress necessary to cause an angina attack can vary from time to time.

_____ 3. The most common symptom of angina is pain.

_____ 4. During an angina attack, the patient moves about a great deal in an effort to get comfortable.

_____ 5. Nitroglycerin should be stored in its original bottle with the cap tightly sealed.

_____ 6. Myocardial infarction pain does not occur in the absence of physical exertion or emotional stress.

_____ 7. Nitroglycerin should be placed sublingually and allowed to dissolve.

_____ 8. Orthostatic hypotension and headache are common side effects of nitroglycerin.

_____ 9. Angina pectoris never advances to myocardial infarction.

_____ 10. Pain associated with myocardial infarction is usually relieved by nitroglycerin.

MEDICAL EMERGENCY!

CASE STUDY 11-1

A 44-year-old male presents with a positive medical history. He indicates on the medical history that he has been experiencing angina attacks for two years. He has his nitroglycerin with him. He is in the office to have an amalgam placed in tooth number 12. The dentist administers anesthesia and begins treatment. The patient becomes pale and starts to clutch at his chest. The dentist stops treatment and allows the patient to administer his own nitroglycerin. The patient says his chest pain is usually not so severe. He tries to get up and move around in an effort to relieve the pain. After several minutes, the patient's pain still has not been relieved. The patient takes another dose of nitroglycerin, but the pain still does not stop.

Questions

1.   Is the patient most likely suffering from angina or myocardial infarction?

2.   What treatment should be followed after administering the second dose of nitroglycerin?

3.   Should oxygen be administered to this patient? Why or why not?

4.   What should the dental assistant be doing during this treatment?

CASE STUDY 11-2

A 64-year-old male presents with a positive medical history. He states that he has had two heart attacks in the last two years. As the dental treatment begins, the dental auxiliary notes that the patient's skin has become cold and clammy. The patient reports a feeling of tightness in his chest.

Questions

1.   Is the patient experiencing angina pectoris or a myocardial infarction? Explain your answer.

2.   What medication should be given to this patient?

3.   List the treatment for this patient's condition.

CHAPTER 12

Cardiopulmonary Resuscitation (CPR)

LEARNING OUTCOMES

Upon completion of this chapter, the student will be able to:

- Explain the CAB guidelines for performing CPR
- Explain the purpose of the automated external defibrillator (AED)
- Demonstrate how to determine consciousness
- Describe the technique for administering rescue breathing
- Demonstrate how to check the carotid pulse
- Explain the technique for administering external compressions
- Explain when CPR should be started and stopped
- Describe the technique of two-person CPR
- Explain how to open the airway in a child or infant
- Explain how to provide rescue breathing for infants and children
- Demonstrate how to check an infant's pulse at the brachial artery
- Explain how to administer external compressions for infants and children
- Describe two of the dangers associated with administering CPR

KEY TERMS

automated external defibrillator (AED)	carotid artery	mandible	stoma
	external compression	pulse	xiphoid process
brachial artery	gastric distention	rescue breathing	
cardiac arrest	laryngectomy	sternum	

The content of this chapter is intended as an overview of the cardiopulmonary resuscitation (CPR) technique. All dental team members should maintain a CPR certification, which is offered by the American Heart Association and the American Red Cross. This certification should be renewed on a regular basis. Keep in mind that advances and modifications in techniques are constantly occurring, so it is important for dental auxiliaries to maintain current certification to ensure they are using the most up-to-date CPR techniques.

CARDIAC ARREST

cardiac arrest When the heart has stopped.

Cardiac arrest exists when the circulation of blood either is absent or is inadequate to maintain life. Although cardiac arrest may be the end result of conditions such as angina or myocardial infarction (discussed in Chapter 11), it also may occur by itself with no previous signs and symptoms of coronary disease.

Cardiac arrest may present as one of three conditions:

1. *Cardiovascular collapse.* The heart is still beating but is so weak that it cannot circulate the blood.
2. *Ventricular fibrillation.* Individual muscles beat independently rather than as a unit, which results in no blood being circulated.
3. *Cardiac standstill.* The heart has stopped beating.

In the past, if a person experienced some form of cardiac arrest, the chances of survival prior to admittance to a hospital were remote. Once the technique of cardiopulmonary resuscitation was devised, these odds were improved. Cardiopulmonary resuscitation, more commonly known as CPR, consists of a combination of external cardiac compressions, establishment of a cardiac rhythm with an automated external defibrillator (AED) in an attempt to force oxygenated blood throughout the body, and rescue breathing.

automated external defibrillator (AED) A portable computerized device that automatically diagnoses a potentially life-threatening cardiac arrhythmia when attached to a pulseless patient.

An **automated external defibrillator** or **AED** is a portable computerized device that automatically diagnoses a potentially life-threatening cardiac arrhythmia when attached to a pulseless patient (see Figure 12-1). The computerized program will analyze the patient's status and determine if an electric shock is necessary. If the electric shock is necessary, the device will give the rescuer instructions on how to proceed. Once the electric shock is delivered, the arrhythmia will cease and allow the heart to reestablish an effective cardiac rhythm.

sternum Narrow, flat bone located at the midline of the thorax.

The effects of CPR are able to be achieved primarily because of the location of the heart. The heart is located between the **sternum** and thoracic spine and is surrounded on either side by the lungs and pericardium. As a result of this location, force applied to the lower sternum creates a pressure that drives the blood through the aorta and pulmonary artery. This blood is then oxygenated by the combination of compressions and rescue breathing.

Since the inception of CPR, those within the medical community have argued about its benefits as well as its hazards. Nevertheless, it has been proven that CPR saves lives. The greatest risk of death from heart attack occurs in the first two hours after the onset of symptoms. If the public is trained in CPR, persons experiencing a heart attack can receive treatment immediately, which increases the chances of survival. As a result of the number

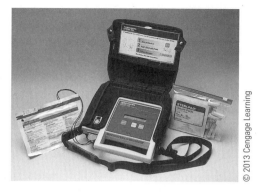

© 2013 Cengage Learning

FIGURE 12-1   Automated external defibrillator (AED).

of people trained in CPR, between 100,000 and 200,000 American lives are saved each year. The biggest advantage of CPR is that it can provide immediate treatment for respiratory arrest or cardiac arrest without the need for any adjunct personnel.

CPR TECHNIQUE

The technique of CPR is broken down into steps known as CAB. The C stands for *chest compressions,* the A for *airway,* and the B for *breathing.* The acronym CAB designates the order in which CPR must be performed (see Emergency Basics 12-1).

Emergency Basics 12-1

CAB Guidelines for CPR

C   Chest compressions
A   Airway
B   Breathing

When a dental patient loses consciousness or is discovered in an unconscious state, the immediate recognition of a cardiac arrest and the activation of the emergency medical services system are essential for the survival of the patient. The presence or absence of circulation must be determined immediately. If circulation is absent, external compression must be combined with defibrillation and rescue breathing, thereby administering full CPR. If breathing is absent, opening the airway and providing rescue breathing may be all that is needed.

Determining Consciousness

The first step of treatment is to determine consciousness. In most dental settings, this is not as difficult as in a public situation because the dental patient is usually being observed when unconsciousness occurs. This step can be accomplished by tapping the patient firmly on the shoulder and shouting in the patient's ear, "Are you all right? Are you all right?" The rescuer must make sure the patient is unconscious and not asleep or in a drug-induced stupor.

Checking the Pulse

pulse The regular expansion and contraction of an artery caused by the ejection of the blood from the left ventricle of the heart as it contracts.

carotid artery Artery located on either side of the neck; used to measure the pulse during an emergency.

The next step is to determine if the patient has a **pulse.** Cardiac arrest is recognized by the absence of a pulse in the large arteries. To determine whether there is a pulse, the rescuer uses the first two fingers of the closest hand to check the person's carotid pulse. (Review the information on vital signs in Chapter 3.)

The **carotid artery** is used to determine the presence of a pulse because it is accessible without removing any clothes, the rescuer is already positioned close to this area, and, most important, there may be a pulse in this artery even when the pulse in the periphery is absent. This artery is located by placing fingers on the person's larynx and sliding them into the groove between the trachea and the muscles on the side of the neck. There is a carotid artery on either side of the neck; either one may be used to check the pulse (Figure 12-2). When checking the pulse, the rescuer should never compress too hard, because the artery could be occluded.

The pulse should always be checked for at least 6 seconds but not more than 10 seconds. It is important to wait at least 6 seconds because in some emergency situations, the pulse may have slowed to such a point that it would not be palpable for at least 6 seconds. If a pulse is present, the rescuer can continue to administer rescue breathing. If a pulse is not present, the rescuer needs to activate the EMS system and retrieve the AED. These actions are completed by instructing another member of the dental team or a bystander, depending on the circumstances, to call 911 for medical help and to retrieve the AED. It is important for the 911 caller to give exact directions to the location so that the emergency team can get to the patient quickly.

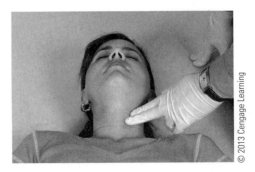

FIGURE 12-2   Location of the carotid artery. The carotid artery is the preferred artery to check for a pulse during a suspected cardiac arrest.

TEST YOUR KNOWLEDGE

1. What is the sequence for CPR?

2. Which artery is the most important to check in an emergency situation such as a suspected cardiac arrest?

EXTERNAL COMPRESSION

external compression
Outside pressure placed on the lower sternum in order to force the blood out of the heart.

Absence of a pulse indicates that the heart is no longer supplying blood and that the blood must be replaced by external compression. **External compression** consists of applying rhythmic pressure over the lower sternum, which raises the thoracic pressure and forces the blood out of the heart. Figure 12-3 demonstrates proper CPR compression technique. Chest compression does not have to be accompanied by rescue breathing. The most recent CPR standards emphasize the importance of high-quality compressions, with adequate rate and depth.

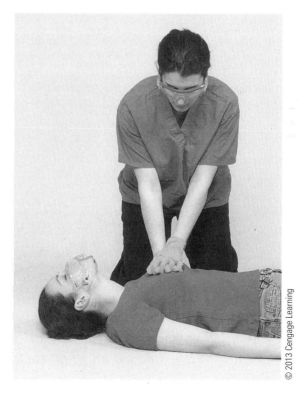

© 2013 Cengage Learning

FIGURE 12-3   Chest compression used during CPR.

Positioning the patient correctly before administering compression is extremely important. The person in cardiac arrest must always be placed in the horizontal position. The external compressions are able to force blood throughout the body, but they are not powerful enough to overcome the forces of gravity in a person who is in any position other than horizontal.

In addition, the patient must be on a firm surface. Since the whole purpose of external compression is to squeeze the heart between the sternum and spine, if the patient is on a soft surface, the force of the compression is absorbed. Contoured dental chairs are not recommended for performing compression. A dental patient who requires compression should be placed either on the floor or on a board inserted between the patient and the chair.

Technique

Once the patient is properly positioned, external compression is administered following these steps:

1. The rescuer is positioned close to the patient's chest.
2. The rescuer must locate the proper hand position for administering the compressions by placing the index and middle finger of the hand closest to the person's feet at the base of the person's rib on the side closest to the rescuer.
3. The rescuer then slides the fingers up the rib cage to the area where the ribs meet the sternum (Figure 12-4).
4. The middle finger rests at this area with the index finger placed beside it. This technique is used to locate the lower portion of the sternum. The location is extremely important because if the hand position is too low, compression takes place over the

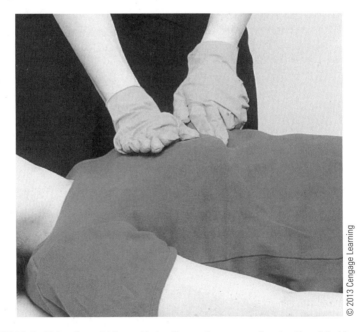

© 2013 Cengage Learning

FIGURE 12-4   Using the middle and index finger, the rescuer locates the xiphoid process and moves up to the lower sternum to begin proper compressions.

xiphoid process Lowest portion of the sternum.

xiphoid process rather than the lower sternum. If compressions are performed over the xiphoid process, it can be broken and the liver can be lacerated; and if compressions are too high, they will be ineffective.

5. Once the lower part of the sternum is located, the heel of the hand closest to the patient's head is placed directly beside the index finger.

6. The first hand is then removed and placed on top of the hand resting on the sternum.

7. The fingers are interlocked, which helps keep the fingers off the chest during compression. Fingers pressing on the chest during compression can damage the ribs.

8. The rescuer's elbows are locked and the shoulders positioned over the hands. This way the compressions are performed by utilizing the rescuer's body weight rather than utilizing only the arm muscles (see Figure 12-3).

9. The size of the patient determines the depth the chest must be compressed to achieve effective compression. For an adult, the sternum is compressed approximately 2.0 inches. This depth is required to adequately force the blood out of the heart.

10. Immediately following the compression, the rescuer releases the sternum to allow the heart to refill. During this release, the hands are not removed from the chest, since correct hand position must not be lost.

11. Compressions should be smooth and rhythmic, with equal time spent on compression and release.

12. In one-person CPR, the rescuer should maintain a ratio of 100 compressions in 60 seconds.

13. After the 30th compression, the rescuer administers two full slow breaths and then returns to the chest, locates the correct hand position, and continues compressions.

14. The AED should be attached and used as soon as it is available. The rescuer should minimize the interruptions in the compressions and resume CPR after each shock or defibrillation.

15. If there is a pulse and breathing, the rescuer monitors the patient. If there is no pulse, the rescuer continues CPR.

TEST YOUR KNOWLEDGE

1. What is the ratio of compressions per breaths in adult CPR for one rescuer?

2. What is the purpose of the automated external defibrillator?

OPENING THE AIRWAY

If rescue breathing is required, it will be necessary to open the airway. After opening the airway, if the patient is not breathing independently, the rescuer will need to breathe for the patient. These two steps combined constitute **rescue breathing.** These steps should be performed after compressions have been started and the emergency medical service system has been activated.

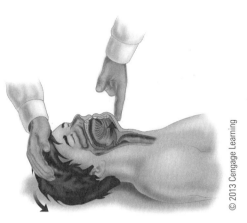

FIGURE 12-5 The head tilt/chin lift technique for opening a patient's airway.

rescue breathing
The act of
assisting or
stimulating
respiration for a
patient who is
not breathing
independently.

mandible Lower
jaw.

When opening the airway, the rescuer should keep in mind that the tongue is the most common cause of airway obstruction in an unconscious person. An individual who loses consciousness may also lose muscle tone, which can cause the tongue to drop to the back of the throat, blocking the airway. Consequently, to open the airway, a method that pulls the tongue away from the back of the throat must be used. This is best achieved by implementing a technique known as the head tilt/chin lift (see Figure 12-5). To accomplish this, the rescuer places the hand closest to the patient's head on the forehead and gently tilts the head back. At the same time, the rescuer uses the hand closest to the patient's feet to lift the patient's chin by placing the fingers—not the thumb—under the bony part of the **mandible** at the chin and lifting the chin upward. This technique lifts the tongue away from the airway. Care must be taken not to close the patient's mouth completely or to put pressure on the soft tissues located under the chin.

Rescue Breathing

To administer rescue breathing, the rescuer first seals the nose by pinching the person's nostrils between the thumb and forefinger of the hand that was on the person's forehead. Next, the rescuer takes a deep breath, opens his or her mouth very wide, and places it around the outside of the person's mouth. If the rescuer's lips are placed on the inside of the person's mouth, a good seal will not form and air will leak around the edges, preventing sufficient air from entering the person's lungs. Once a good seal has formed, the rescuer blows air into the person's mouth. During the ventilations, the rescuer should observe the person to make sure sufficient oxygen is reaching the person's lungs. This can be achieved by watching the rise and fall of the chest, feeling slight resistance as the air enters the person's lungs, and feeling the air escape during exhalation.

If the rescuer is able to get air into the person's lungs, the first breathing sequence should consist of two breaths with 1 to 1.5 seconds allowed for each breath. Each breath should be separate, allowing the lungs to deflate between each breath.

A rescuer who is unable to get air into the person's lungs should reposition the airway and attempt to ventilate again. If it is still impossible to get air into the lungs, the rescuer must assume there is an airway obstruction and should follow the procedures covered in Chapter 10.

Mouth-to-Nose Respiration Some conditions require that respiration be administered using a mouth-to-nose technique rather than a mouth-to-mouth technique. For example, this may be necessary when the mouth is damaged to such an extent that a good seal cannot be formed. If this technique is required, the rescuer should keep the head tilted back with the hand on the forehead and use the other hand to close the person's mouth. The rescuer then makes a seal with the mouth around the person's nose and administers the two slow breaths.

laryngectomy
Excision of the larynx.

Mouth-to-Stoma Respiration As treatment for certain conditions, some persons may have had a **laryngectomy.** This results in a **stoma,** or opening, that connects the trachea directly to an opening in the skin. In these situations, it is necessary for the rescuer to administer ventilations directly to the person's stoma. It is not necessary to open the airway because the stoma is at the bottom of the airway.

stoma A small opening.

Gastric Distention When the rescuer is administering rescue breathing, a condition known as **gastric distention** can occur. This condition is seen most frequently in children, although it can also occur in adults. Gastric distention usually occurs when the rescuer uses too much air to ventilate the person or when the airway is partially or completely blocked, which forces air into the stomach rather than the lungs.

gastric distention
Enlargement of the stomach due to an increase of air being forced into it; usually seen as a result of forceful rescue breathing.

Severe gastric distention can be dangerous because it may cause regurgitation with the vomitus aspirated into the lungs, causing an obstruction. Furthermore, it can reduce the lung capacity if the distended stomach causes the diaphragm to be elevated.

STARTING AND STOPPING CPR

To achieve the greatest benefits, CPR should be started immediately upon recognition of cardiac arrest. Some degree of brain damage may occur if the brain is deprived of oxygen for more than six minutes; if CPR is not started within this time, it is unlikely that the patient will be restored to previous central nervous system (CNS) levels. If the rescuer is not certain the person is experiencing cardiac arrest, the person should receive the benefit of the doubt and the rescuer should attempt CPR. Once CPR has been started in the absence of a physician, it should be continued until one of the following conditions is met:

1. The person recovers.
2. CPR efforts are transferred to another qualified person trained in CPR.
3. A physician assumes responsibility for the person.

4. EMS personnel (EMTs or paramedics) assume responsibility for the person.
5. The rescuer is exhausted and physically unable to continue CPR.

See Emergency Basics 12-2 for the rates and rhythms used when one person is performing CPR.

Emergency Basics 12-2

One-Person CPR

Hand position: 2 hands
Rates: 30 compressions, 2 breaths
Depth: 2.0 inches

TWO-PERSON CPR

The rates and rhythms previously covered apply to one-person CPR for adults. Although CPR can successfully be performed by one rescuer, it quickly becomes physically exhausting when a single person must carry out compressions and respirations. It is much more beneficial if two people can work together to perform CPR. Two-person CPR consists of one person administering compression while the second person administers respiration.

If two rescuers begin CPR together, one person is positioned at the person's chest and is responsible for administering compression while the second person is positioned at the head and is responsible for maintaining an open airway and providing respiration. The second rescuer can retrieve the AED as well as notify EMS personnel. There may be situations when one person is alone and must begin CPR, but a second person can join the first rescuer on arrival.

TEST YOUR KNOWLEDGE

1. Under what conditions can a rescuer stop administering CPR?

2. Why must a rescuer have a good seal when administering rescue breathing?

CPR FOR INFANTS AND CHILDREN

Cardiac arrest does not occur very often in infants or children. Nevertheless, there may be some emergency situations when cardiac arrest occurs and CPR is required. The basic principles of CPR are the same for adults, infants, and children. However, the anatomical differences in size require a few adjustments in techniques.

Categorizing Infants and Children

For purposes of CPR, an infant is considered anyone under one year of age. A child is anyone between one and eight years of age. Anyone over eight is treated as an adult. In some individuals where actual age is unknown, size may make it difficult to determine whether the individual should be treated as a child or an infant. There should be no delay in starting CPR in an effort to determine if the person is a child or an infant, as a slight error one way or the other will not cause a major problem.

Determining Consciousness in the Infant or Child

When an infant or child with a problem is discovered, it is necessary to first determine consciousness. The tap-and-shout method discussed for adults is also appropriate for a child, but a slightly different technique may be more beneficial with an infant. Sometimes it is difficult to tap an infant with enough force to assume unconsciousness while still being gentle enough to prevent injury. Therefore, to determine consciousness in an infant, the rescuer should thump the bottom of the infant's foot while shouting the baby's name, if it is known. If there is no response to these stimuli, the rescuer should assume the infant is unconscious.

Positioning the Infant/Child

Once the rescuer determines that an infant or child is unconscious, the next step is to position the person. Whether a child or an infant, the person should be placed supine on a hard flat surface. When dealing with an infant, better access may be provided by placing the infant on a table or countertop rather than on the floor.

External Compressions

Child When administering compressions for a child, the first step is to locate the correct hand position, achieved the same way as for adults. The bone structure of a child is more fragile than that of an adult, so the same amount of force is not needed to compress the sternum. Only the heel of one hand is used to compress the sternum 2.0 inches.

The rate of compressions per minute for a child is 100. The ratio of breaths per compression is 30:2 for a single rescuer and 15:2 for two rescuers.

Infant An infant's heart is located considerably higher in the chest than an adult's; the hand position for an infant is located at the midsternum right between the two nipples. The bone structure of an infant is even more delicate than a child's. Therefore, only the index and middle fingers of one hand are used to compress the midsternum 1.5 inches.

The rate of compressions per minute for an infant is 100. The ratio of breaths per compression is 30:2 for a single rescuer and 15:2 for two rescuers.

Automated External Defibrillation (AED)

To use an AED with pediatric patients, the rescuer must use an AED that is calibrated for use with infants and children. The electrical dose for defibrillation is not precisely known, but the use of relatively high doses of energy has not resulted in any adverse effects.

Opening the Airway

After the infant or child is properly positioned, the rescuer opens the airway. For this process, the head tilt/chin lift technique may be used. The technique should be performed the same as for adults except that it is extremely important not to overextend the child's or infant's neck when tilting the head. This could damage the neck as well as close the airway instead of opening it.

Checking for Air Exchange

The rescuer must then check to see if the infant or child is breathing. This can be done by placing an ear close to the person's mouth, looking for the rise and fall of the chest, listening for air exchange, and feeling for air against the cheek.

Breathing

If the infant or child is not breathing, the rescuer must provide rescue breathing. The technique for rescue breathing varies for infants and children:

- *Child.* If the child is large enough for the rescuer to form a good seal around the mouth, the air may be provided using the same techniques as with the adult. If the child is smaller than that, the rescuer will need to use the infant technique.

- *Infant.* In the case of an infant or a very small child, the rescuer needs to form a seal by placing the mouth over the infant's mouth and nose.

Once a sufficient seal is achieved by covering the mouth or mouth and nose, the rescuer should administer two full slow breaths.

Remember that the lungs of infants and children are smaller than an adult's, so the amount of air administered must be adjusted according to the size of the child. The air passages of the infant and child are also smaller, and as a result provide more resistance when the rescuer attempts to blow air into the person's lungs. The rescuer should not be afraid to use some force to get air into the lungs.

If the rescuer is unable to get air into the lungs of the child or infant, the airway should be reopened and an attempt made to ventilate again. If it is still impossible to get air into the person's lungs, the rescuer should assume there is an airway obstruction and proceed as described in Chapter 10. On the other hand, if air flows easily into the person's lungs, the rescuer should provide the two full slow breaths and proceed to the next step.

Checking the Pulse

The next step in the CPR sequence is to check the pulse of the infant or child. In a child, the presence of a pulse can be determined by palpating the carotid artery. In an infant,

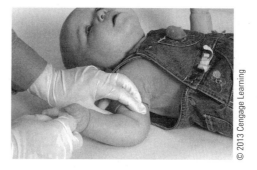

FIGURE 12-6   The brachial artery is the most effective way to detect a pulse on an infant.

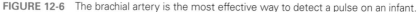

brachial artery
The principal
artery of the
upper arm.

however, it is sometimes difficult or even impossible to palpate the carotid artery because an infant usually has a very short, fat neck that prevents access to that artery. Therefore, it is best to check the infant's pulse by palpating the **brachial artery.** The brachial artery is located on the inside of the arm midway between the elbow and the shoulder (Figure 12-6). To palpate this pulse, the rescuer places the thumb on the outside of the infant's arm and the index and middle finger over the brachial artery and presses, lightly. Some people have difficulty locating this pulse, and extra practice should be directed to this area when mastering CPR skills.

If a pulse is present but breathing is absent, the rescuer should provide rescue breathing only, utilizing the following rates:

- *Infant.* One puff every 3 seconds
- *Child.* One breath every 4 seconds

If the brachial or carotid artery is palpated and there is no pulse, the rescuer must provide external compressions.

DANGERS OF CPR

Because of the location of the ribs, sternum, and other organs, as well as the force required to perform CPR, injuries to the patient may occur. Incorrect hand position or excessive force can result in broken ribs. Placing the hands too low on the sternum and compressing the xiphoid process can lacerate the liver. Any of these factors can cause major problems to the person, but should never cause the rescuer to hesitate in beginning CPR.

SUMMARY

Thousands of Americans die from cardiac arrest each year. Some of these deaths occur in the dental office. By mastering the skills of CPR, the auxiliary puts forth a concerted effort to save lives, both in the dental setting and in everyday life.

REVIEW QUESTIONS

MULTIPLE CHOICE

1. Which of the following components comprise CPR?
   (1) rescue breathing
   (2) external compression
   (3) checking blood pressure
   (4) administering nitroglycerin
      a. 1, 2, 3
      b. 2, 3
      c. 1, 2
      d. 3, 4

2. Put the following steps of CPR in the correct order.
   (1) place the AED
   (2) administer external compressions
   (3) open airway
   (4) activate EMS system
      a. 1, 2, 3, 4
      b. 3, 1, 4, 2
      c. 4, 2, 1, 3
      d. 2, 1, 3, 4

3. Which of the following techniques should be used to administer ventilations to a person who has had a laryngectomy?
      a. mouth-to-stoma
      b. mouth-to-mouth
      c. mouth-to-nose
      d. none of the above

4. When performing CPR on an adult, the _____ artery should be checked to determine the presence of a pulse.
      a. brachial
      b. radial
      c. femoral
      d. carotid

5. For an adult, external compressions should be administered
      a. at midsternum.
      b. over the xiphoid process.
      c. over the lower half of the sternum.
      d. none of the above

6. On an adult, the sternum should be compressed
   a. 1.0 inch.
   b. 2.5 inches.
   c. 1.5 inches.
   d. 2.0 inches.

7. On an adult, the ratio of compressions to breaths is
   a. 15 compressions: 2 breaths.
   b. 30 compressions: 2 breaths.
   c. 15 compressions: 1 breath.
   d. none of the above

8. When checking the pulse on an infant, the _____ artery should be used.
   a. brachial
   b. femoral
   c. carotid
   d. radial

9. On a child, the sternum should be compressed
   a. 2.0 inches.
   b. 1.0 inch.
   c. 1.5 inches.
   d. 2.5 inches.

10. When administering compressions for an infant, the rescuer should use
    a. both hands interlocked.
    b. the index and middle fingers of one hand.
    c. the heel of one hand.
    d. none of the above

TRUE OR FALSE

_____ 1. The biggest advantage of CPR is that is can be started immediately without any additional personnel.

_____ 2. The shock from an AED is used to stop the heart muscle from defibrillating.

_____ 3. Gastric distention will never cause any problems for the person.

_____ 4. For an infant, the correct hand position is determined by following the ribs up to the lower part of the sternum.

_____ 5. When administering rescue breathing for a person who has had a laryngectomy, the rescuer will administer respirations over the person's mouth and nose.

_____ 6. For an adult, compressions and respirations are administered at a rate of 15:2.

_____ 7. Once CPR has been started, the rescuer may stop if he or she feels that the person is not responding.

_____ 8. During two-person CPR, one rescuer provides rescue breathing while the other rescuer provides compressions.

_____ 9. The tap-and-shout method may be used on a child to determine consciousness.

_____ 10. There are no dangers to people who have CPR performed on them.

MEDICAL EMERGENCY!

CASE STUDY 12-1

A 40-year-old male presents with a negative medical history. His appointment is for a regular six-month dental checkup. While the appointment is in progress, the patient begins to complain of tightness in his chest. He clutches his chest and then loses consciousness. The rescuer utilizes the head tilt/chin left technique to open the airway. The rescuer then checks for breathing and determines that the patient is not breathing. The rescuer gives one breath and then locates the brachial artery to determine if the person has a pulse. No pulse is found, so the rescuer telephones the EMS system for help. Next, the rescuer locates the lower half of the sternum and uses the heel of one hand to compress the sternum 1.5 inches. The rescuer administers 15 compressions, then returns to the person's head and administers two breaths. After 10 or 12 cycles, the rescuer decides the patient is not responding and stops CPR.

Questions

1. List all the errors in this procedure.

2. For each error listed, explain what technique should have been used.

CASE STUDY 12-2

A 52-year-old male presents with a positive medical history. He reports on his medical history that he is taking medication for a heart condition and hypertension. As the dental auxiliary prepares for the procedure, the patient begins to complain of chest pains and loses consciousness. The dental auxiliary notifies the dentist and the receptionist and begins chest compressions. Once the dentist enters the operatory, she places a hard backboard under the patient and prepares the AED. The receptionist notifies the EMS system and retrieves the emergency kit.

Questions

1.   What steps should be done next?

2.   Why is it important to retrieve the AED?

3.   What would the ratio of compressions to breaths be for this patient?

SECTION FIVE

Immune System Emergencies

This section deals with localized and systemic medical conditions and emergencies that involve the immune system.

CHAPTER 13: Allergic Reactions

CHAPTER 13

Allergic Reactions

LEARNING OUTCOMES

Upon completion of this chapter, the student will be able to:

- Describe the functions of the immunoglobulin system
- Explain what must take place for an allergic reaction to occur
- Explain the special importance of a thorough medical history when dealing with an allergic patient
- Explain the signs, symptoms, and treatment for allergic skin reactions
- Define an anaphylactic reaction
- Describe the signs and symptoms associated with an anaphylactic reaction
- Explain the treatment for an anaphylactic reaction with allergic symptoms
- Explain the treatment for an anaphylactic reaction without allergic symptoms
- Describe the role of epinephrine in treating allergic reactions
- Describe the steps to follow when a patient is allergic to dental anesthesia
- Explain the signs and symptoms associated with latex allergy
- Describe the protocol to follow when a staff member or patient is allergic to latex

KEY TERMS

anaphylaxis	cardiac arrhythmias	histamine	shock
angioedema	contact dermatitis	immune system	urticaria
antibody	edema	immunoglobulin system	vesicle
antigen	erythema	latex allergy	

A 45-year-old female has an appointment with the dentist to have a class I amalgam placed in tooth number 20. Upon examining her medical history, the auxiliary notes that the patient is in excellent health except for listing allergies to dust, penicillin, sulfur drugs, insect stings, and seafood. The dentist administers the anesthesia, and within 30 seconds the patient begins to exhibit problems. She complains that it feels as if her throat is closing; she is nauseated, itches all over, and is becoming very anxious. The dentist diagnoses acute anaphylactic reaction. The auxiliary immediately transmits the epinephrine-loaded syringe to the dentist. Once the medication is administered by the dentist, the patient begins to recover. This patient was experiencing a severe anaphylactic reaction to the anesthesia. Without proper treatment, she would have died within minutes.

A vast majority of the population is allergic to one thing or another. The reaction to this allergy may range from a slight rash and runny nose to a fatal anaphylactoid reaction. To understand an allergic reaction, it is important to understand the functions and makeup of the body's **immune system.**

immune system A biological complex that protects the body against pathogenic organisms and other foreign bodies.

ANTIBODIES

antibody A protein produced to react specifically with an antigen.

immunoglobulin system Five structurally and antigenically distinct antibodies present in the serum and external secretions of the body.

An **antibody,** which is produced by the lymphoid tissues, is an essential part of the body's immune system. Antibodies are produced when a virus, bacteria, or some other foreign substance enters the body. A particular type of antibody is produced for each foreign substance, which is called an *allergen* or *antigen.* So far, five different classifications of antibodies have been discovered. Together they make up the **immunoglobulin system.** Refer to Figure 13-1.

Immunoglobulin A (IgA) antibodies are found in areas of the body such as the nose, breathing passages, digestive tract, ears, eyes, and vagina. IgA antibodies protect body surfaces that are exposed to outside foreign substances. This type of antibody is also found in saliva, tears, and blood. IgA is found in all the secretions of the body and helps protect the body from dangerous microorganisms.

Immunoglobulin D (IgD) antibodies are found in small amounts in the tissues that line the belly or chest and in serum tissue. The precise function of the IgD antibody has not been determined.

Immunoglobulin E (IgE) antibodies are found in the lungs, skin, and mucous membranes. They cause the body to react against foreign substances such as pollen, fungus spores, and animal dander. They may occur in allergic reactions to milk, some medicines,

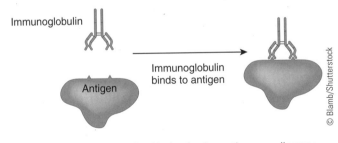

FIGURE 13-1   Immunoglobin antibodies bind to foreign antigens or allergens.

and some poisons. IgE antibody levels are often high in people with allergies and are responsible for reacting with certain antigens and causing type I reactions, which are anaphylactic reactions.

Immunoglobulin G (IgG) antibodies are found in all body fluids. They are the smallest but most common antibody. IgG antibodies are very important in fighting bacterial and viral infections. IgG antibodies are the only type of antibody that can cross the placenta in a pregnant woman to help protect her baby (fetus).

Immunoglobulin M (IgM) antibodies are the largest antibody. They are found in blood and lymph fluid and are the first type of antibody made in response to an infection or exposure to a foreign antigen.

See Emergency Basics 13-1 for a summary of the antibodies that make up the immunoglobulin system.

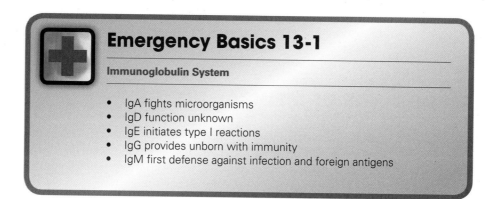

Emergency Basics 13-1

Immunoglobulin System

- IgA fights microorganisms
- IgD function unknown
- IgE initiates type I reactions
- IgG provides unborn with immunity
- IgM first defense against infection and foreign antigens

ANTIGENS

antigen
Substance that causes the formation of an antibody; also known as *allergen*.

An **antigen**, sometimes called an *allergen,* is a substance that enters the body and can produce a hypersensitive reaction but is not necessarily intrinsically harmful. Most people develop a natural or acquired immunity to allergens, but in people who suffer from allergies, the body is overly sensitive to the antigen. When an allergic reaction occurs, the body's immune system is not protecting itself against the allergen.

ALLERGIC REACTIONS

When an antigen enters a body, the body's defense mechanism goes into play. Basic defense mechanisms such as the skin, the lining of the nasal passages, and other first-line-of-defense mechanisms attempt to block the antigen from entering the system. If this does not work and the antigen enters the system, the immunoglobulin system goes into action.

In most cases the antigen is destroyed. If for some reason the antigen is not destroyed, biochemicals may be released, which can result in various degrees of allergic reaction.

Prerequisites for Reactions

histamine
Substance normally found in the body; its functions include increasing gastric secretions, constriction of the smooth muscles of the bronchioles, and dilation of capillaries.

A person does not experience an allergic reaction during the first exposure to the antigen. For example, a person who is going to be allergic to penicillin does not experience any reaction the first time the drug is given. This first dose is known as the sensitizing dose. After this dose, the body produces the IgE antibody, which reacts only to this particular antigen. For a period after exposure, the IgE antibody continues to be produced while the antigen decreases. After a certain time, only the specific IgE antibody is circulating in the body. At this point no allergic reaction occurs.

When the person is exposed again to this same allergen, or one that is chemically similar, an allergic reaction does occur. This results as the body recognizes the antigen, and biochemical elements that cause the reaction are released. The main biochemical element is **histamine.** Histamine is found in all cells but is only released in allergic reactions. It has the ability to cause dilation of the capillaries, increased secretion of the gastric juices, decreased blood pressure, and constriction of some of the smooth muscles. The type of allergic reaction that results depends mainly on the type and amount of allergen involved.

IMPORTANCE OF MEDICAL HISTORY

The medical history is especially important when dealing with an allergy-prone patient. It has been determined that a person with a history of allergies to several substances (such as pollen, eggs, seafood, and penicillin) is very likely to experience an allergic reaction to some item or drug used in the dental office. Evidently this person's body responses are highly sensitized, and the patient requires special attention during the dental procedures.

In addition, the medical history is important in telling the dental staff what substances have actually caused the patient to experience an allergic reaction. For example, if a patient reports experience in the past of an allergic reaction to xylocaine, the dental team would not use this particular drug during the procedure.

TEST YOUR KNOWLEDGE

1. What is the immunoglobulin that is responsible for causing type I reactions?

2. What are the effects of histamine on the patient's tissue?

3. What is the most important item that a dental auxiliary can obtain from a patient that will prevent allergic reactions?

TYPES OF ALLERGIC REACTIONS

Allergic reactions vary in type and severity. The reaction may occur almost immediately because of the humoral system or may be delayed for several days as a result of the cell-mediated system. The reaction may be localized to one area, such as a skin reaction, or may be generalized, involving the whole body, as in an anaphylactoid reaction. Refer to Figure 13-2.

In some instances it is possible to predetermine the severity of a reaction. The time that elapses between exposure to the allergen and the onset of the allergic reaction determines to a great extent the severity of the reaction. If some reaction is noticed within a few minutes of exposure, the reaction may be much more severe than when the reaction is seen several hours to a few days after the exposure.

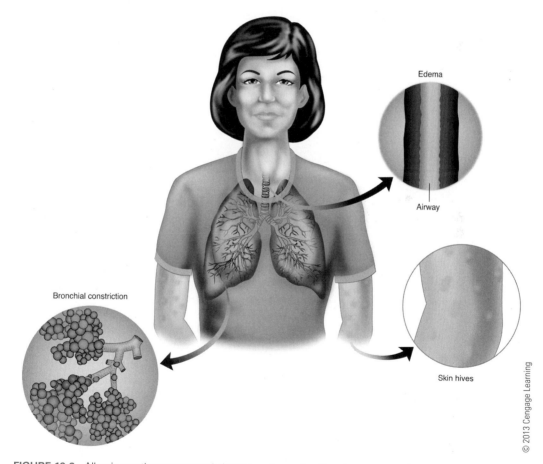

Edema

Airway

Bronchial constriction

Skin hives

© 2013 Cengage Learning

FIGURE 13-2   Allergic reactions vary greatly in type and severity. Reactions can manifest in a range from skin reactions, such as urticaria (commonly known as hives), to extreme cases such as laryngeal edema (swelling of the larynx) due to an anaphylactic allergic reaction. All allergic reactions require prompt treatment.

Skin Reactions

contact dermatitis Inflammation of the skin from contact with a sensitizing agent.

erythema Redness of the skin.

edema Local or generalized swelling from retention of excessive fluid.

vesicle An elevation of the epidermis containing fluid; also known as a *blister*.

There is a wide variety of skin disorders, ranging from mild to very severe. Skin reactions may also be the first stage of anaphylactoid reactions. So, no matter how mild it seems, the progression of a skin reaction should be watched carefully.

Contact Dermatitis Contact dermatitis is an allergic skin reaction that occurs as a result of cutaneous exposure to a particular allergen and may occur in the oral mucosa as well as in the skin. The allergen that causes this type of reaction may include such items as poison ivy, toothpaste, mouthwash, lipstick or other cosmetics, impression materials, metal alloys, and stainless steel wire. Contact dermatitis is usually an acute problem, but if the allergen is not removed and exposure continues, the condition becomes chronic and in some cases disabling.

The first signs of contact dermatitis include **erythema** (redness), **edema** (swelling), and **vesicle** (blister) formation. In some intense cases these vesicles may rupture and result in open, oozing wounds. The main symptom is intense itching. This symptom, as well as the condition, is usually localized to the one area where the antigen contacted the surface, although in a few cases it may spread.

In most cases, the first step of treatment is to remove the contacting substance. A physician may further administer corticosteroids and antihistamines.

See Emergency Basics 13-2 for a summary of the signs/symptoms and treatment of contact dermatitis.

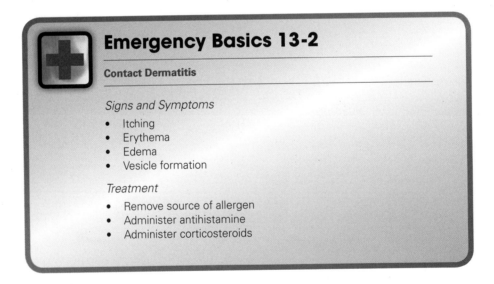

Emergency Basics 13-2

Contact Dermatitis

Signs and Symptoms
- Itching
- Erythema
- Edema
- Vesicle formation

Treatment
- Remove source of allergen
- Administer antihistamine
- Administer corticosteroids

urticaria A skin reaction characterized by the eruption of itching wheals; also known as *hives*.

Urticaria Urticaria is a skin condition most of the general public calls hives (see Figure 13-2). It may be caused by any substance that is either ingested or placed on the skin surface. This condition consists of circumscribed raised areas of erythema and edema, and as with any allergic reaction, it may be mild or severe.

As with contact dermatitis, the main course of treatment is to remove the substance. The patient may be given instructions to take an over-the-counter antihistamine. If the symptoms persist, the patient may need to contact his or her physician. For example, if the urticaria was caused by some substance that the patient ingested, the course of treatment would be to stop the ingestion of the substance.

See Emergency Basics 13-3 for a summary of the signs/symptoms and treatment of urticaria.

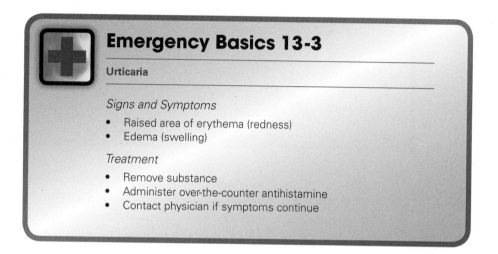

Emergency Basics 13-3

Urticaria

Signs and Symptoms
- Raised area of erythema (redness)
- Edema (swelling)

Treatment
- Remove substance
- Administer over-the-counter antihistamine
- Contact physician if symptoms continue

angioedema An allergic reaction characterized by swelling of the skin or mucous membrane.

Angioedema In its beginning stages, **angioedema**, also called *angioneurotic edema*, is sometimes mistaken for urticaria. Basically, angioedema is a giant form of urticaria. It is characterized by localized swelling of either the submucosa or subcutaneous tissues. The lesions associated with angioedema have certain characteristics: usually the lesions are single, but in some cases they may be multiple; they are very large and do not have defined raised borders like urticaria; and there is no pain and usually no associated itching. The tissues of the genitals, face, and hands are the areas usually affected by angioedema.

Angioedema is usually caused by an allergic reaction to drugs, food, or environmental factors. As with most skin reactions, angioedema occurs when an antigen enters the body, histamine is released, capillaries dilate, and fluid enters the area. It is commonly seen in people with a history of various allergies but may also be found in those with no allergy history.

Treatment consists of removing the cause and administering an antihistamine. In most cases this treatment reverses the situation without major complications occurring. However, if the incident takes place in the dental office, the dental team should watch the patient carefully for a period of time to make sure the swelling does not increase in an area in which it may potentially interfere with respiration.

See Emergency Basics 13-4 for a summary of the signs/symptoms and treatment of angioedema.

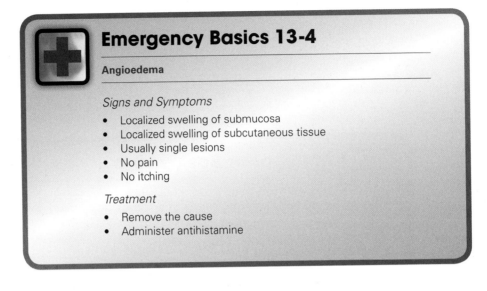

Emergency Basics 13-4

Angioedema

Signs and Symptoms

- Localized swelling of submucosa
- Localized swelling of subcutaneous tissue
- Usually single lesions
- No pain
- No itching

Treatment

- Remove the cause
- Administer antihistamine

Note that in most mild cases of allergic skin reactions, the dentist may choose not to treat the patient in the dental office but rather refer the patient to a physician or allergist. This action may prove satisfactory, but the dental team should observe the patient and always provide follow-up treatment either in the office or by referral.

Most skin reactions do not create emergency situations in themselves. The major cause for concern is that skin reactions may either advance and create an emergency or be the beginning of a true emergency situation such as anaphylactic shock.

TEST YOUR KNOWLEDGE

1. Which type of allergic reaction occurs as a result of direct exposure to an allergen?

2. What areas of the body are most often affected by angioedema?

3. In general, what is the treatment for most allergic reactions in a dental office?

Respiratory Allergic Reactions

Allergic reactions that may affect only the respiratory system also occur. The most common type of respiratory reaction, asthma, is covered in detail in Chapter 8.

ANAPHYLACTIC REACTION

anaphylaxis
A severe life-threatening allergic reaction.

An anaphylactic reaction is a severe allergic reaction that occurs in previously sensitized patients. It develops almost immediately after the patient ingests, inhales, or is injected with an antigen or is stung by an insect. **Anaphylaxis** is the most severe allergic reaction and often proves fatal regardless of the treatment administered.

Physiology

As with other allergic reactions, anaphylaxis occurs only in those who have been previously exposed to the allergen. The patient is exposed to the allergen, an incubation period then takes place, and antibodies form. When the patient is exposed to the same allergen, the anaphylactic reaction occurs. This is sometimes called the exciting or shock dose, which is how the name anaphylactic shock came into existence.

Severity

Symptoms associated with anaphylaxis can vary in a wide range of severity that depends on the amount of acquired sensitivity, the amount of antigen that entered the body, and the method in which the antigen entered the body. Furthermore, the time that elapses between the exposure to the antigen and the onset of symptoms usually indicates how serious the reaction will be. For example, reactions that occur within the first 30 minutes after contact with the antigen are usually the most severe. Reactions that occur after 30 minutes are less likely to be fatal.

Symptoms

Signs and symptoms associated with anaphylaxis vary in both type and severity. These may be seen in the skin, gastrointestinal, respiratory, or circulatory systems. A common term used to describe these signs and symptoms is **shock.**

shock A life-threatening condition that occurs when the body is not getting enough blood flow.

Shock is best described by a decrease in perfusion of oxygenated blood to the organs in the body. This condition can be the result of a physical trauma or, in the case of allergies, a release of chemicals that diminish the ability of the cardiac and pulmonary systems to supply oxygenated blood. As a result, the organs of the body begin to fail and toxins are produced that increase the signs and symptoms reported in a patient experiencing shock.

Signs and symptoms associated with the skin in allergic reactions may include generalized pruritus (itching), urticaria, or angioedema. Normally these conditions are not too dangerous, but they do have the potential to become life-threatening if they are located in some specific areas. For example, angioedema located around the mouth or throat could cause death from airway obstruction. Gastrointestinal signs and symptoms may include varying degrees of nausea, vomiting, and diarrhea.

Respiratory signs and symptoms may include varying degrees of airway obstruction. This most often occurs as a result of laryngeal edema, a swelling of the larynx that occurs as a result of an allergic reaction (see Figure 13-2). The swelling may be great enough to cause partial or even complete obstruction of the airway. It is the most common cause of death in anaphylactic reactions.

cardiac arrhythmias
Abnormal rhythms of the heart.

Circulatory signs and symptoms may include hypotension, shock, **cardiac arrhythmias,** and even complete circulatory collapse.

All the signs and symptoms associated with an anaphylactic reaction vary in their severity as well as in the way they present themselves. Nevertheless, diagnosis can be relatively easy if the signs and symptoms occur right after the exposure. In this situation, almost immediately the patient will feel faint and weak, will begin sweating, and will become anxious and restless. The patient then develops a severe itching sensation as a result of allergic skin reactions. The condition then proceeds through the gastrointestinal, respiratory, and circulatory stages. If this cycle is not stopped, the end result will be death.

See Emergency Basics 13-5 for a summary of the signs and symptoms of anaphylaxis.

Emergency Basics 13-5

Signs and Symptoms of Anaphylaxis

Skin
- Generalized pruritus (itching)
- Urticaria
- Angioedema

Gastrointestinal
- Nausea
- Vomiting
- Diarrhea

Respiratory
- Laryngeal edema

Circulatory
- Hypotension
- Shock
- Cardiac arrhythmias
- Complete circulatory collapse

Additional Symptoms
- Sweating
- Anxious feeling
- Nervousness

One distinct problem associated with anaphylactic shock is that, in some cases, the reaction can be so severe that all the signs and symptoms occur at once. In these situations diagnosis may be more difficult, and death may occur regardless of any treatment.

Treatment

At the very first sign of an anaphylactic reaction, place the patient in a supine position and administer oxygen. The receptionist should summon emergency medical assistance. In the meantime, the dental auxiliary should retrieve the emergency kit and prepare an epinephrine injection; the dentist should administer the epinephrine immediately. Remember that a subsequent injection of epinephrine may be required. If more than one injection of epinephrine is needed, the dentist may administer an injection of antihistamine during the acute phase.

During the entire episode, attention must be paid to the patient's airway, since laryngeal edema may cause the airway to become blocked. However, once the epinephrine is administered, the patient's condition should improve. If laryngeal edema occurs and complete airway obstruction results, the dental auxiliary should be prepared to assist the dentist in performing a cricothyrotomy. If there is a complete loss of blood pressure and/or pulse, the dentist and auxiliary should begin CPR until medical assistance arrives.

The treatment just described is specific for an anaphylactic reaction that demonstrates the signs and symptoms mentioned earlier. But as stated earlier, a unique problem with the anaphylactic reaction is that, in some cases, the reaction is so severe that the signs and symptoms occur quickly and seem to happen all at once. In this situation, the patient may become unconscious almost immediately, and it may be difficult to determine that the condition was caused by an allergic reaction.

When there are no definitive signs of an allergic reaction, the dentist should not administer epinephrine. Instead the patient should be placed in the Trendelenburg position, basic life support provided as needed with extra attention paid to maintaining the airway, and emergency medical assistance summoned. If the condition worsens, CPR or cricothyrotomy may become necessary.

The dental team can administer oxygen to a patient suspected of having an allergic reaction. Oxygen administered through a nasal cannula or face mask will not harm the patient or make the reaction worse.

See Emergency Basics 13-6 for a summary of the treatment of anaphylaxis both for patients with obvious signs and symptoms and for patients in whom it is not clear whether an allergic reaction has caused the condition.

EPINEPHRINE

In the treatment of severe allergic reactions, epinephrine is the drug of choice. Epinephrine is a vasopressor, has antihistaminic action, and is a bronchodilator (Figure 13-3). Its effect is extremely rapid in onset. This characteristic in particular makes it especially useful in the treatment of anaphylactic reactions when time is crucial.

Emergency Basics 13-6

Treatment of Anaphylaxis

Patient with Obvious Signs and Symptoms

1. Summon medical assistance
2. Place the patient in a supine position
3. Administer oxygen
4. Administer epinephrine
5. Administer antihistamine as needed
6. Initiate CPR if needed
7. Assist dentist in performing cricothyrotomy if necessary

Patient Without Signs or Symptoms

1. Summon medical assistance
2. Do not administer epinephrine
3. Place patient in Trendelenburg position
4. Provide basic life support as needed
5. Administer oxygen
6. Initiate CPR if needed
7. Assist dentist in performing cricothyrotomy if necessary

Although epinephrine is extremely beneficial in the treatment of allergic reactions, it should never be administered unless you are sure the patient is suffering from an allergic reaction. Some conditions, such as cerebrovascular accident, may at first be mistaken for an allergic reaction, since the patient may lose consciousness. In such situations, administering epinephrine, which increases blood pressure, could cause extreme harm.

TEST YOUR KNOWLEDGE

1. What is the most common cause of death in a patient exhibiting signs of anaphylaxis?

2. Why should a dentist not administer epinephrine to a patient without being certain that the patient is experiencing an allergic reaction?

3. What is meant by the term *shock*?

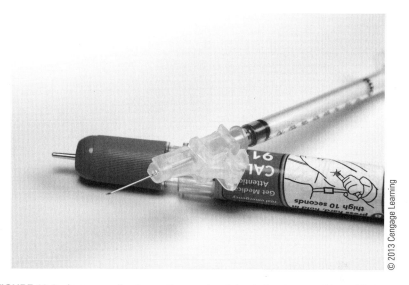

© 2013 Cengage Learning

FIGURE 13-3   In severe allergic reactions, epinephrine is the drug used to rapidly reverse the symptoms of anaphylactic shock. It is of utmost importance to confirm that the patient is suffering an allergic reaction, and not another medical emergency, before administering epinephrine.

ALLERGY TO ANESTHESIA

One aspect of allergic reactions unique to dentistry is an allergic reaction to dental anesthetic solutions. However, if a patient reports an allergy to dental anesthesia on the medical history, the dentist should explore the subject a little further. Many patients are denied treatment with anesthesia because they have been told they are allergic to anesthesia when actually their reaction was not an allergic one at all, but a result of some other problem. It has been estimated that less than 1 percent of all negative reactions to anesthesia are actually allergic reactions.

Nevertheless, there are cases in which the patient is actually allergic to the anesthesia and will indeed experience an allergic reaction. The majority of reactions are characterized by inflammation, papules, edema, and pruritus. The response can be severe enough to cause an anaphylactic reaction. These reactions should be treated according to the appropriate section on treatment earlier in the chapter. Luckily, patients who are allergic to one type of anesthesia can sometimes be given anesthesia from another chemical group to which they are not allergic.

LATEX ALLERGIES

latex allergy A medical term encompassing a range of allergic reactions to natural rubber latex.

Allergy to natural rubber latex is now recognized as an increasingly serious medical problem that affects not only health care workers, but also the general population. The incidence of **latex allergies** has increased dramatically since the 1980s. Allergic reactions to latex can range from minor skin irritations to fatal anaphylactic reactions. Because the minor skin reactions mimic so many common situations, they are often overlooked by the individual or even misdiagnosed by physicians.

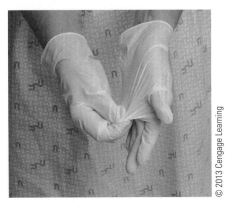

FIGURE 13-4   Latex allergies can develop at any time, especially in those who work with latex on a consistent basis, like dental auxiliaries.

Individuals at Risk

Both individuals with a genetic history of allergies and individuals with a high exposure to latex products are at an increased risk for latex hypersensitivity. In these instances, the risk tends to increase with greater exposure (see Figure 13-4). Some studies have stated that 8 to 12 percent of health care workers with regular exposure to latex are sensitized, as compared to 1 to 6 percent of the general public. These percentages, especially with regard to health care workers, continue to increase.

Additional risk factors may include a history of surgery, disorders requiring repeated urinary catheterization, and certain food allergies including bananas, avocados, chestnuts, and kiwi. See Emergency Basics 13-7 for a list of individuals who are at high risk for latex allergies.

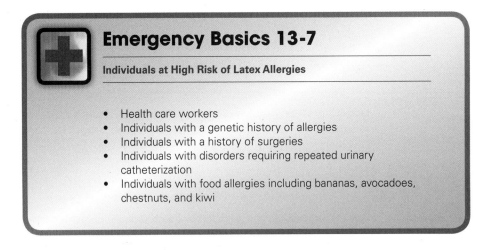

Emergency Basics 13-7

Individuals at High Risk of Latex Allergies

- Health care workers
- Individuals with a genetic history of allergies
- Individuals with a history of surgeries
- Individuals with disorders requiring repeated urinary catheterization
- Individuals with food allergies including bananas, avocadoes, chestnuts, and kiwi

Although a high incidence of latex allergies occurs in health care workers, a dental office must be prepared to deal with patients with this same allergy.

Signs and Symptoms

Three different types of reactions may be seen in individuals who are allergic to latex (see Emergency Basics 13-8). The two most common reactions from exposure to latex products are contact dermatitis or a delayed contact reaction. Contact dermatitis may result in dry, itchy, irritated areas of the skin, usually the hands. A delayed contact reaction is very similar to a poison ivy reaction. It typically occurs 48 to 72 hours after exposure and may include a red, itchy rash or possibly blisters.

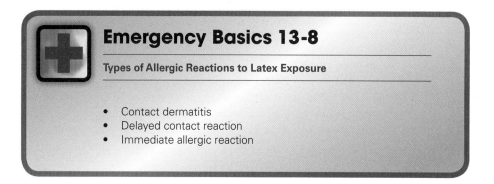

Emergency Basics 13-8

Types of Allergic Reactions to Latex Exposure

- Contact dermatitis
- Delayed contact reaction
- Immediate allergic reaction

The third type of reaction to latex exposure is the immediate allergic reaction. The signs of this reaction usually occur 2 to 3 minutes after contact with the latex. In this situation, the individual may experience itching at the area of contact followed by welts or rash. These signs may disappear within 30 minutes. Additional immediate reactions may occur in individuals with sensitivity to airborne allergens associated with latex. This is commonly associated with powder used with latex gloves. This powder can be released as a result of putting on or removing gloves as well as by removing gloves from the glove box. The latex particles attach themselves to the powder and become airborne. As a result, sensitized individuals may experience coughing, wheezing, shortness of breath, and respiratory distress. The severity of the reaction depends on the sensitivity of the individual. In extreme cases, where sensitivity is extremely high, an anaphylactic reaction may occur.

Treatment

Currently there is no cure for latex allergy. Prevention and avoidance of exposure to latex and treatment of symptoms are the main treatment options.

Should one of the three types of allergic reactions to latex exposure occur in a staff member or a patient, the treatment discussed in the previous sections of this chapter should be provided.

Prevention

Individuals must be tested by a physician to determine that they have a true allergy to latex. In individuals in which a true latex allergy has been diagnosed, protocols should be taken to prevent or minimize exposure to latex.

In order to minimize exposure to latex, sensitized dental staff members should:

- Use nonlatex gloves and products
- Learn to recognize the signs and symptoms of latex allergy
- Avoid areas where powder from latex gloves worn by others might be inhaled
- Inform employer and staff of the allergy
- Wear a medical alert bracelet

When treating a patient who indicates a diagnosed allergy to latex, the following steps should be implemented:

- When possible, schedule this person as the first patient of the day
- Do not use latex products in the treatment room
- Prepare/set up the treatment room with nonlatex gloves
- Handle instruments with nonlatex gloves
- Wear nonlatex gloves during treatment
- Use latex-free materials and instruments

New information on latex allergies continues to be developed. New products that are latex-free enter the market on a daily basis. All dental professionals should continue to seek education on this topic and make changes as more information becomes available.

SUMMARY

Allergic reactions in the dental office can be fatal. The amount of treatment the auxiliary is allowed to perform, although not lacking in importance, is somewhat limited. Since the main method of treatment in severe reactions is an injection of epinephrine, the treatment must be performed by the dentist. It is nevertheless very important for the auxiliary to understand what takes place during a reaction and assist the dentist by having all drugs prepared. Remember, in an anaphylactic reaction, death can occur quickly if correct treatment is not provided. The auxiliary should also help the dentist administer CPR if this becomes necessary. A competent and calm team will make the treatment progress efficiently and professionally, which will benefit the well-being and health of the patient.

REVIEW QUESTIONS

MULTIPLE CHOICE

1. The immunoglobulin responsible for causing type I allergic reactions is
   a. IgA.
   b. IgE.
   c. IgG.
   d. IgM.

2. The foreign substance that enters the body and causes an allergic reactions is a/an
    a. antibody.
    b. lymph cell.
    c. immunoglobulin.
    d. antigen.

3. An allergic skin reaction that occurs as a result of direct exposure of the skin to a/an
    particular allergen is
    a. contact dermatitis.
    b. angioedema.
    c. urticaria.
    d. laryngeal edema.

4. An allergic skin reaction that is also known as hives is
    a. contact dermatitis.
    b. angioedema.
    c. urticaria.
    d. laryngeal edema.

5. The treatment for angioedema consists of
    a. removing the cause.
    b. administering an antibiotic.
    c. administering an antihistamine.
    d. a and c

6. The most common type of allergic respiratory reaction is
    a. emphysema.
    b. bronchitis.
    c. tuberculosis.
    d. none of the above

7. The most important part of treating an anaphylactic reaction consists of administering
    a. oxygen.
    b. antihistamine.
    c. corticosteroid.
    d. epinephrine.

8. The most common cause of death associated with an anaphylactic reaction is
    a. hypotension.
    b. laryngeal edema.
    c. cardiovascular collapse.
    d. none of the above

9. Which of the following is a function of histamine?
    a. dilation of the capillaries
    b. secretion of gastric juices
    c. decreased blood pressure
    d. all the above

10. Which of the following areas of the body are most often affected by angioedema?
    (1) torso
    (2) hands
    (3) face
    (4) genitals
        a. 1, 2, 3, 4
        b. 1, 2, 4
        c. 2, 3, 4
        d. 2, 3

TRUE OR FALSE

_____   1. A patient who is allergic to one type of dental anesthesia may be able to tolerate another type.

_____   2. A patient usually experiences an allergic reaction on first exposure to the harmful antigen.

_____   3. The time that elapses between exposure to an antigen and the onset of symptoms helps in determining the severity of the upcoming reaction.

_____   4. The patient with a history of allergies to several things is a likely candidate for an allergic reaction in the dental office.

_____   5. The main symptom of contact dermatitis is swelling.

_____   6. It is not uncommon for a person to die from a severe anaphylactic reaction even if proper treatment is provided.

_____   7. Signs and symptoms associated with an anaphylactic reaction may be seen in the skin, gastrointestinal, respiratory, or circulatory system.

_____   8. The signs and symptoms of an anaphylactic reaction never occur so rapidly that they cannot be distinguished.

_____   9. A dentist who is not sure the patient is suffering from an anaphylactic reaction should not administer epinephrine.

_____   10. Patients who state they once experienced an allergic reaction to dental anesthesia should be checked out by an allergist.

MEDICAL EMERGENCY!

CASE STUDY 13-1

An 18-year-old male presents with a negative medical history. He has an appointment with the dentist for the extraction of the upper-right third molar. The dentist enters the operatory and administers the injection of anesthesia. In less than a minute the patient loses consciousness. There are no signs or symptoms of an allergy.

Questions

1.   What should be the first step in treating this patient?

2.   Should epinephrine be administered?

3.   Should medical help be summoned?

CASE STUDY 13-2

A 21-year-old male presents with a negative medical history and reports to be in good general health. The treatment planned for today is a tooth-colored restoration on a maxillary first molar. As the auxiliary is placing a latex dental dam, the patient begins to complain of itching around his lips. No previous reaction has been noted in the treatment record.

Questions

1.   What is the most likely cause of the itching?

2.   What should be the first step in treating this patient?

3.   What notation should be placed in the patient's medical history update?

SECTION SIX

Legal Issues in Emergency Care

This section deals with the legal issues that are a part of emergency treatment.

CHAPTER 14

Occupational Hazards and Emergencies

LEARNING OUTCOMES

Upon completion of this chapter, the student will be able to:

- Explain the hazards of mercury contamination
- Explain how to prevent mercury contamination
- Describe how to avoid the hazards of ionizing radiation
- Describe universal precautions and PPE
- Describe how to prevent breakage of an anesthetic needle
- Explain the treatment needed to remove a broken endodontic file or reamer
- Explain how the auxiliary can help prevent soft-tissue injuries
- Describe ways to prevent the patient from aspirating foreign objects
- Describe the hazards of nitrous oxide/oxygen conscious sedation

KEY TERMS

endodontic file

endodontic reamer

ionizing radiation

personal protective
  equipment (PPE)

universal precautions

Most emergencies in the dental office occur as a result of some associated medical condition. However, some emergencies occur as a result of the dental treatment itself, and there are conditions in the dental office that present hazards to the dental personnel as well.

The first section of this chapter covers hazards present in the dental office that have the potential to injure office personnel. The second section presents a few of the more common emergencies that can arise as a result of certain dental procedures.

HAZARDS TO OFFICE PERSONNEL

A number of potential hazards can directly or indirectly affect the dental auxiliary. However, when hazardous conditions or materials are treated with care, most of these hazards can be eliminated or rendered harmless.

Mercury Contamination

The use of amalgam as a restorative material has diminished as a result of the improvement of tooth-colored restorative materials. However, amalgam still remains as a restorative material because of its strength and durability. Since one of the major components of amalgam is mercury, the dental auxiliary should be aware of the potentially toxic effects of mercury poisoning. Although mercury has potential for causing serious problems within the dental office, if handled properly, it need not be an occupational hazard.

Mercury can be absorbed through the skin if the auxiliary handles it improperly during the preparation of amalgam. However, mercury is absorbed mainly by inhalation of vapors in the air. Mercury vapors can be released into the air by improperly storing scrap amalgam, by spilling mercury in the operatory, and by removing a worn or broken amalgam restoration with a high-speed handpiece without water.

Mercury poisoning can cause birth defects, brain dysfunction, kidney problems, and other associated conditions. In addition, mercury poisoning is extremely dangerous because the dental team may never be aware that an office is contaminated until serious effects have taken place.

The protocols for mercury hygiene should be an important consideration for the dental team. To prevent mercury poisoning, the following precautions should be taken:

1. Never touch the amalgam or mercury with bare hands.
2. Enclose scrap amalgam in a tight container with used x-ray fixer or a specially prepared mercury solution that can be purchased from most supply companies. (At one time it was suggested that scrap amalgam be stored in water, but we now know that water does not prevent the emission of mercury vapors.)
3. Try to prevent all mercury spills. If a spill does occur, special techniques should be followed. Always use one of the several devices that can be purchased for the purpose of collecting a spill. Never collect a mercury spill with the high-volume evacuation system or a vacuum cleaner.
4. When removing a worn or broken amalgam restoration, always use water with the high-speed handpiece. The high-volume evacuator suction tip should always be placed close to the operative site to catch any debris or dust removed from the tooth.
5. Most state governmental agencies have departments that will come into the dental office to monitor mercury levels upon request. This should be done on a routine basis.

TEST YOUR KNOWLEDGE

1. How can the dental team reduce the chances of mercury contamination?

2. How should scrap amalgam be stored to prevent vapors from being released?

Radiation

Dental radiation, when used properly, is one of the most beneficial diagnostic tools available, but when used carelessly, it is a potential occupational hazard. The damaging effects of **ionizing radiation** are widely known. Some auxiliaries, however, are not aware of the situations that place them in danger of being exposed to excessive amounts of radiation.

ionizing radiation
High-energy electromagnetic waves such as x-rays.

To prevent radiation exposure, the auxiliary should:

1. The dental auxiliary should always stand behind a lead-lined shield to prevent any exposure to the ionizing radiation.
2. Always be at least six feet away from the x-ray head, which will place the technician out of the range of the x-ray beam.
3. Never hold the film in the patient's mouth.
4. Wear a personal monitoring device. This usually takes the form of a film badge that monitors the amounts of radiation to which an auxiliary is exposed (see Figure 14-1). These may be purchased through several different companies. The badges are returned each month to the company, which monitors and reports the amount of radiation exposure, if any.

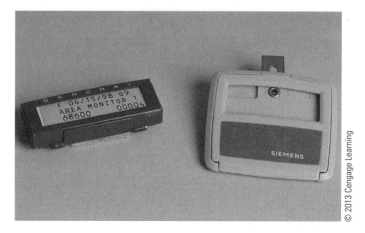

© 2013 Cengage Learning

FIGURE 14-1   Film badges should be worn to monitor radiation exposure.

Biological Hazards

universal precautions
Approaches and protocols adopted to protect health care workers and their patients from getting and spreading disease and infection.

The dental auxiliary is exposed to biological blood-borne or saliva-borne pathogens, ranging from HIV to hepatitis to herpes simplex. The standard of care in contemporary dental offices is to treat each patient with **universal precautions**, meaning that all patients are treated as if they are infectious. The hazard of exposure to biological pathogens is minimized by the use of **personal protective equipment (PPE)**. Personal protective equipment includes, but is not limited to, the following:

- Protective eyewear (i.e., goggles, dental face shield; see Figure 14-2a)
- Gloves (i.e., latex, vinyl, etc.; see Figure 14-2b)
- Masks (see Figure 14-2c)
- Protective clothing (i.e., dental auxiliary gown or uniform)

If there is a breakdown in the infection control standards, the auxiliary may be exposed to a biological hazard. In this situation, the dental auxiliary will need to follow the protocols mandated by the office, clinic, or institution that employs the auxiliary.

(A)

(B)

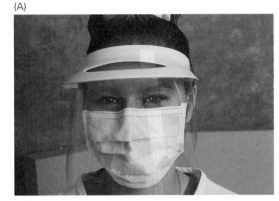
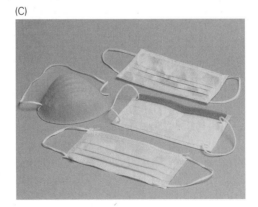

(C)

© 2013 Cengage Learning

FIGURE 14-2 Examples of personal protective equipment commonly used in the dental office: (A) dental face shield; (B) vinyl and latex gloves; (C) face masks.

personal protective equipment (PPE) Protective clothing and equipment, such as face shields and gloves, used in occupations to protect workers from injury and infection.

TEST YOUR KNOWLEDGE

1. When should the dental auxiliary hold a radiographic film in the patient's mouth?

2. What are some examples of PPEs?

PATIENT DENTAL EMERGENCIES

This section describes some of the emergency situations that may occur in the office as a result of dental treatment. Many dentistry-related emergencies can occur, but this section is limited to those that seem to occur most often.

Broken Anesthetic Needle

An anesthetic needle may be broken during an injection because of poor technique by the dentist, a needle imperfection, or an abrupt violent movement by the patient. This kind of emergency occurs more often during a mandibular injection because of the position of the needle. The auxiliary can help prevent this emergency by examining the needle before the injection and by keeping the patient from grabbing or hitting the dentist's hand during the injection.

If this emergency should occur, the patient should be informed of the situation by the dentist. The auxiliary should do everything possible to help keep the patient calm. Removal of a broken needle can be a complicated surgical procedure. Therefore, unless the dentist has extensive surgical experience, he or she usually refers the patient to an oral surgeon. The auxiliary should record the entire incident in the patient's chart. This may prove valuable should later legal action be taken.

Separated Endodontic Reamer or File

endodontic file or reamer A dental instrument used to remove the contents of the pulp chamber.

During endodontic therapy, an **endodontic file** or **reamer** may separate and remain in the root canal of the tooth. To prevent further complications, the dentist must remove this fragment. The auxiliary must be prepared to assist with any procedure the dentist chooses.

Soft-Tissue Injury

During surgical procedures, it is extremely common for the surgical site to become very slippery, and consequently it is easy for a sharp surgical instrument to slip off the tooth and lacerate the surrounding soft tissues. This may wound the tongue, cheek, or gingival areas. The dentist will treat each such area as required, and the auxiliary should be prepared to assist with any necessary procedure.

In some situations, the auxiliary can help to prevent laceration of the soft tissue by providing proficient suctioning, which keeps the area clear and increases visibility. The auxiliary also can use a mirror or other instrument to retract the tongue from the surgical area.

TEST YOUR KNOWLEDGE

1. How can the dental auxiliary prevent an anesthetic needle from breaking?

2. Why is the potential for soft tissue injury present during dental procedures?

Aspiration of a Foreign Object

The dental office is the perfect setting for the aspiration of an object into the airway. The patient is supine, the saliva makes everything slippery, and the dental team is constantly placing small objects in and removing them from the patient's mouth. A few common objects aspirated by patients include crowns, bridges, dental-dam clamps, and burs. The auxiliary can play an important role in preventing the aspiration of small objects by taking the following preventive steps.

When trying in crowns, whether permanent or temporary, the auxiliary should unfold a 2 × 2 gauze and place it across the back of the throat, in front of the gag-reflex area, as a screen. If the crown is dropped, it will be caught in the gauze and can be easily removed. Similarly, a 2 × 2 gauze should be in place when teeth are being extracted to catch any pieces that may break. If the dentist is trying in a bridge, the auxiliary should tie a 10- to 12-inch piece of floss around the pontic and hold onto the end of the floss while the dentist tries in the bridge.

When placing a dental-dam clamp, the auxiliary should tie a piece of floss around the clamp and hold the floss while the clamp is placed on the tooth. If the clamp slips off the tooth, the auxiliary will be holding the floss and it will not be aspirated.

A dental bur can break at any time and a small part could be aspirated. This may be prevented by utilizing a dental dam whenever possible. Furthermore, the auxiliary should always tug on the bur before it is used to make sure it is firmly placed in the handpiece.

Nitrous Oxide/Oxygen Conscious Sedation

Nitrous oxide/oxygen conscious sedation is being used with increasing frequency in today's dental office. When used properly, it provides a more pleasant experience for most anxious dental patients. On the other hand, if used incorrectly, nitrous oxide/oxygen conscious sedation can become a hazard not only to the patient but also to the dental team.

During recent years, it has become known that continuous exposure to nitrous oxide/oxygen vapors can be hazardous to dental personnel. When nitrous oxide/oxygen conscious sedation is administered through a nosepiece, some amount of the gas leaks around the mask. In the past, the dental team was constantly inhaling these escaping vapors. Physical problems such as miscarriages and infertility have been noted to occur as a result of this exposure. Today's units have an attachment (known as a scavenger unit) that collects any excess gas. All units are required to have this attachment.

When administered at the proper dose and rate, nitrous oxide/oxygen conscious sedation provides a very good sedative for the dental patient. However, if the dosage is incorrect, the substance becomes a general anesthetic and the patient loses consciousness, presenting a serious condition in the dental office that should always be avoided.

To achieve optimal effects from nitrous oxide/oxygen conscious sedation, the dental team must properly explain its effects to the patient. The gas should then be introduced slowly. The dental team should keep constant conversation going during the beginning stages. Uncommunicative patients can suddenly become excited and have been known to injure themselves or dental personnel by unexpectedly jumping out of the chair. In addition, the patient receiving nitrous oxide/oxygen in too high a dosage may begin to vomit, which can create a potential problem if the patient aspirates the vomitus.

Nitrous oxide/oxygen conscious sedation, when administered and monitored properly, can be used safely and effectively. However, the auxiliary should be aware that there are potential complications associated with the use of this form of sedation.

SUMMARY

The dental office can present both the dental team and the patient with hazardous situations. The auxiliary should realize that most of these situations may be prevented if proper precautions are taken. However, no matter what prevention techniques are employed, some emergencies will occur. It is these situations that the auxiliary needs to know how to handle properly.

REVIEW QUESTIONS

MULTIPLE CHOICE

1. Which of the following is not true concerning the handling of mercury?
    a. It should never be touched with the hands.
    b. Scrap amalgam or mercury should be stored in a dry container.
    c. Water spray should be used when removing an old amalgam.
    d. Excess mercury should never be suctioned with the high-volume suction.

2. If the auxiliary must be in the room when the x-ray is being exposed, the auxillary should be
   a. at the patient's feet.
   b. behind a lead screen.
   c. holding the tube head.
   d. all the above

3. The auxiliary may prevent the breaking of an anesthetic needle by
   a. using a larger-gauge needle.
   b. keeping the patient from hitting the dentist's hands.
   c. using a shorter needle.
   d. all the above

4. For optimum protection from infectious diseases, the auxiliary should
   a. wear a mask.
   b. wear gloves.
   c. wear safety glasses.
   d. all the above

5. To eliminate constant exposure to nitrous oxide/oxygen vapors, the dental team should use a unit that has a
   a. scavenger unit.
   b. full-mouth mask.
   c. clear nosepiece.
   d. none of the above

TRUE OR FALSE

_____ 1. Broken anesthetic needles occur most often during maxillary injections.

_____ 2. A broken endodontic file does not need to be removed from the canal.

_____ 3. A 2 × 2 gauze should be placed at the back of the throat to prevent a crown from going down the throat during cementation.

_____ 4. A scavenger unit is not needed on today's nitrous oxide/oxygen conscious sedation units.

MEDICAL EMERGENCY!

CASE STUDY 14-1

A 35-year-old female presents with a negative medical history. The treatment plan for today is to have a crown placed on tooth number 3. The crown has been delivered from the lab and the dentist is preparing to try the crown on the tooth.

Questions

1. Describe what steps should be taken to prevent a possible airway obstruction from occurring during the try-in of the crown.

CASE STUDY 14-2

A 48-year-old male presents with a negative medical history. The treatment plan for today's appointment is to complete an endodontic procedure on tooth number 14. As treatment progresses, a small portion of an endodontic file breaks off in the canal of the tooth.

Questions

1. How should this situation be handled to reduce the risk to the patient and dental team?

CHAPTER 15

Legal Problems of Emergency Care

LEARNING OUTCOMES

Upon completion of this chapter, the student will be able to:

- Explain the dental team's general legal duties to the patient
- Explain ways the dental team can prevent lawsuits against the dental team

KEY TERMS

abandonment   negligence

This chapter is designed to provide the dental auxiliary with very basic information concerning legal problems associated with emergency care. Laws vary from state to state, and auxiliaries should check the laws pertaining to the state of their employment. Furthermore, laws that could affect the outcome of a particular legal action are changing every day, so it is important to stay up-to-date in this area.

DUTIES AND RESPONSIBIITIES

negligence The omission of duty that results in injury or harm to another person.

The number of lawsuits against health professionals is growing. To reduce the risk of such a case, the dental team must first understand its legal obligations to the patient. A failure of the dental team to meet any of its legal duties leaves the team liable for a lawsuit based mainly on **negligence.**

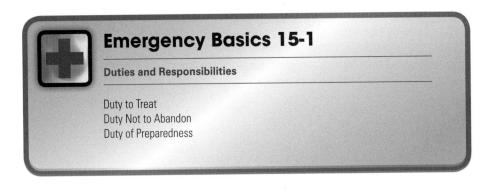

Emergency Basics 15-1

Duties and Responsibilities

Duty to Treat
Duty Not to Abandon
Duty of Preparedness

Duty to Treat

The dental team has an obligation, once it begins treatment, to provide all the treatment required by the patient. In an emergency, the dental team must do everything in its power to provide care for the patient. This treatment requirement also includes the transfer of the patient to a hospital if the scope of the emergency requires more extensive care than that available in the dental office.

Duty Not to Abandon

Once the dental team begins to treat the patient, it has a duty not to abandon the patient. In an emergency situation, this means the dentist must first stabilize the patient and then transfer the patient to a medical facility if necessary. If the dental team did not begin treatment on the patient but merely summoned transportation to a medical facility, the patient may have grounds for legal action. Furthermore, the dental team must never allow the patient to leave the dental office until the emergency is over. For example, if a patient complains of chest pain, is allowed by the dental team to leave while still experiencing the pain, and subsequently experiences a myocardial infarction,

abandonment
Wrongful cessation of the provision of care to a patient.

it is extremely possible that the patient can sue the dental team for negligence on the grounds of **abandonment**.

Duty of Preparedness

The dental team has a legal duty to the patient to be prepared for an emergency. First, the dental team must have the knowledge to administer basic care in the event of an emergency. Second, the office must contain basic emergency equipment such as an oxygen tank and a complete emergency kit. Third, the dentist must have a staff trained in basic emergency treatment.

The dentist is ultimately responsible for the actions of employees while they are at work. However, dental auxiliaries can still be held liable for their actions and included in any lawsuit against the dentist. Auxiliaries therefore have the legal obligation to be prepared for an emergency by being trained in emergency treatment such as CPR.

GOOD SAMARITAN LAW

Most states have enacted Good Samaritan laws. These laws, which give legal protection to people who provide emergency care to ill or injured people, have been developed to encourage people to help others in emergency situations. They require that the "Good Samaritan" use common sense and a reasonable level of skill, and not exceed the scope of the individual's training in emergency situations. They assume that each person will do his or her best to save a life or prevent further injury.

People are rarely sued for helping in an emergency. However, the existence of Good Samaritan laws does not mean that someone cannot be sued in that situation. In rare court cases, courts have ruled that these laws did not apply where an individual rescuer's actions were grossly or willfully negligent or reckless or where the rescuer abandoned the victim after initiating care.

Dental office staff should always be current in their CPR and emergency training and be prepared to assist a patient in the event of an emergency.

TEST YOUR KNOWLEDGE

1. Which member of the dental team is ultimately responsible for the actions of the entire dental team?

2. Can a dental team be liable for not finishing treatment for a patient? Why or why not?

PREVENTING LEGAL PROBLEMS

The dental team cannot prevent every emergency. Similarly, the dental team cannot prevent a patient from bringing legal action. However, the dental team can do several things to prevent the patient from being successful if there is litigation.

First, the dental team must do everything possible to prevent an emergency from occurring. This can be achieved by utilizing optimum, updated dental techniques; by maintaining updated medical histories; and by having the necessary knowledge and equipment to handle an emergency.

Second, the dental team should establish an emergency routine and practice it on a regular basis. This demonstrates that the team is prepared and also enables the team to act more efficiently and effectively during an emergency.

Third, the dental office should have all emergency numbers available near the phone. One office member should be designated to summon medical assistance when needed.

Finally, should an emergency occur, the auxiliary should write down, in detail, everything that transpired prior to, during, and after the emergency. This will prove extremely important if a patient sues, enabling the defense to present the court with the pertinent facts of the emergency.

SUMMARY

Patients can initiate lawsuits against any member of the dental team. Each state's legal requirements for the dental team differ. It is important for the dental team to be aware of its responsibilities. By being aware of those responsibilities, the dental team will be better prepared to prevent legal actions or to answer them.

REVIEW QUESTIONS

MULTIPLE CHOICE

1. The law that gives legal protection to people who provide emergency care to ill or injured people is
   a. ADAA Code of Ethics.
   b. Americans with Disabilities Act.
   c. Good Samaritan Law.
   d. HIPAA.

2. Which of the following is not a general legal duty to the patient?
   a. not to abandon
   b. preparedness
   c. treat
   d. none of the above

3. A patient experiencing documented chest pains is allowed to leave the dental office still experiencing chest pains. The patient can sue the dental team based on what grounds of legal duty?
   a. abandonment
   b. ethics
   c. preparedness
   d. none of the above

4. Which of the following is/are necessary to fulfill the legal duty of preparedness in a dental office?
   a. basic emergency equipment
   b. knowledge to administer basic life support
   c. training in basic emergency treatment
   d. all of the above

5. Who is ultimately responsible for the actions that occur in the dental office?
   a. dental office manager
   b. dental auxiliary
   c. dentist
   d. receptionist

TRUE/FALSE

_____ 1. The dental staff does not have to have current CPR and emergency training.

_____ 2. A failure of a dental team to meet any of its legal duties leaves the team liable for a lawsuit.

_____ 3. The laws pertaining to emergency treatment are the same in each state.

_____ 4. Negligence occurs if the dental team fails to meet any of its legal duties.

MEDICAL EMERGENCY!

CASE STUDY 15-1

A 45-year-old female presents with a negative medical history. She has come to the dental office for a checkup and cleaning. During the appointment, the patient experiences chest pains. The dental team determines that the patient is possibly experiencing a heart attack. They provide treatment for the patient and call for emergency medical assistance. The patient is transported to the hospital.

Questions

1.   What should the dental team do once the patient is stabilized and transported to the hospital? Why?

CASE STUDY 15-2

A 32-year-old male presents with a negative medical history. He is returning for his last appointment for restorative treatment. During the appointment, the dentist notes that the patient has developed several more dental lesions and informs the patient that he will need to return to complete his treatment. The patient leaves without making another appointment. Several months lapse, and the dentist receives notification that the patient is suing the dentist for abandonment.

Questions

1.   Is the dentist liable for abandonment? Why or why not?

Glossary

A

abandonment Wrongful cessation of the provision of care to a patient.

abdominal thrusts Technique used as part of the Heimlich maneuver, which uses abdominal thrusts to try to dislodge an object.

absence (petit mal) seizure An epileptic seizure characterized by a sudden momentary loss of consciousness occasionally accompanied by minor twitching.

allergen Any substance capable of inducing an allergic reaction.

American Society of Anesthesiologists (ASA) An association of physicians, primarily anesthesiologists, who share a common goal of improving patient care through education and research.

ampule Sealed glass container that holds a single dose of medication.

amyl nitrite A vasodilator.

anaphylaxis A severe life-threatening allergic reaction.

aneurysm Abnormality of a blood vessel, usually an artery, caused most often by a defect or weakness of the vessel wall.

angina pectoris A severe pain in and around the heart caused by an insufficient supply of oxygenated blood to the heart.

angioedema An allergic reaction characterized by swelling of the skin or mucous membrane.

antecubital fossa Area approximately one inch from the elbow at which the stethoscope is placed in order to hear the pulse when measuring blood pressure.

antibody A protein produced to react specifically with an antigen.

antigen Substance that causes the formation of an antibody; also known as an *allergen*.

aorta Main artery of the human body.

arteriosclerosis Thickening of the artery walls that results in loss of elasticity.

ASA Physical Status Classification System A six-category physical status classification system for assessing a patient's risk before treatment; usually the dental team deals with only the first four categories.

asphyxiation Death caused by lack of oxygen.

aspirate To breathe in forcefully causing an object to become lodged in the airway.

assessment Consists of reviewing the medical history and the likely side effects of any prescribed medications.

atherosclerosis Form of arteriosclerosis that affects the coronary arteries and causes coronary artery disease.

atria Upper chambers of the heart.

atrioventricular valve A valve in the heart through which blood flows from the atria to the ventricles.

aura A sight, sound, or smell unique to an individual before experiencing an epileptic seizure.

automated external defibrillator (AED) A portable computerized device that automatically diagnoses a potentially life-threatening cardiac arrhythmia when attached to a pulseless patient.

B

baseline vital signs Vital signs (e.g., blood pressure, pulse, respiration rate, and temperature) that are recorded prior to treatment to help determine how the patient is responding during treatment.

blood pressure   The pressure the blood exerts on the walls of the arteries, the veins, and the chambers of the heart.

brachial artery   The principal artery of the upper arm.

bronchodilator   A medication that dilates the bronchioles.

C

carbon dioxide   A colorless, odorless gas produced by the oxidation of carbon.

cardiac arrest   When the heart has stopped.

cardiac arrhythmias   Abnormal rhythms of the heart.

carotid artery   Artery located on either side of the neck; used to measure the pulse during an emergency.

cerebral infarction   A type of CVA that occurs as a result of some problem in the arterial blood supply from the heart to the brain.

clonic   Movements marked by contraction and relaxation of muscle that are associated with a tonic-clonic (grand mal) seizure.

contact dermatitis   Inflammation of the skin from contact with a sensitizing agent.

coronary artery disease   A condition in which the walls of the coronary arteries become thick and hard.

cranium   The part of the skull that houses the brain.

cyanosis   Bluish skin color that results from decreased oxygen.

D

demand-valve resuscitator   Attachment for the oxygen tank that can force oxygen into the lungs of a nonbreathing victim.

dental dam   A thin sheet of latex or nonlatex rubber for isolating one or more teeth during a dental procedure.

diabetic coma   A life-threatening condition caused by a lack of insulin in the body.

diastolic pressure   Pressure on the arteries when the heart relaxes between beats.

diazepam   A medication used to treat active seizures; also used to treat anxiety, nervousness, and muscle spasms.

Dilantin gingival hyperplasia   Overgrowth of gingival tissue that results from the intake of Dilantin.

E

edema   Local or generalized swelling from retention of excessive fluid.

embolism   A clot that forms somewhere in the body and travels throughout the body until it lodges.

emergency kit   A kit containing the necessary medications and equipment required to treat an emergency.

endocardium   Lining of the inner heart surface.

endodontic file   A dental instrument used to remove the contents of the pulp chamber.

endodontic reamer   A dental instrument used to remove the contents of the pulp chamber.

epicardium   Inner layer of the pericardium.

epigastrium   Area of the upper abdomen.

epilepsy   A type of seizure disorder that affects people for a variety of reasons and is not selective as to ethnicity, age, or gender.

epinephrine   A vasoconstrictor.

erythema   Redness of the skin.

external compression   Outside pressure placed on the lower sternum in order to force the blood out of the heart.

extrinsic asthma   A form of asthma caused by the exposure of the bronchial mucosa to an inhaled airborne antigen. Also may be known as allergic asthma.

F

flowmeter   Attachment on the oxygen tank that controls the amount of oxygen that is delivered to the patient.

G

gastric distention   Enlargement of the stomach due to an increase of air being forced into it; usually seen as a result of forceful artificial respiration.

gestational diabetes   Diabetes that usually occurs first during pregnancy.

glucagon A hormone produced in the pancreas that raises blood sugar.

glucose Fuel for the body manufactured from the food one eats.

H

HbA1C A lab test that shows the average amount of glucose in blood over a three-month period.

Health Insurance Portability and Accountability Act (HIPAA) Signed into law in 1996, a portion of this act establishes rules and regulations that define how information obtained from a patient can be circulated and to whom such information can be distributed with a patient's written consent.

Heimlich maneuver Technique used to remove an object that is lodged in the airway.

hemiplegia Paralysis of one side of the body.

hemorrhage A great amount of blood loss in a short period of time.

histamine Substance normally found in the body; its functions include increasing gastric secretions, constriction of the smooth muscles of the bronchioles, and dilation of capillaries.

hyperglycemia A condition that occurs when there is too much glucose in the blood.

hypertension Abnormally high pressure of the blood against the arterial walls; commonly known as *high blood pressure*

hypoglycemia A condition that occurs as a result of too little glucose in the body.

I

immune system A biological complex that protects the body against pathogenic organisms and other foreign bodies.

immunoglobulin system Five structurally and antigenically distinct antibodies present in the serum and external secretions of the body.

insulin Hormone secreted by the pancreas.

insulin shock A life-threatening condition caused by an excess of insulin in the body.

intrinsic asthma A nonallergic form of asthma usually first occurring later in life that tends to be chronic and persistent rather than episodic. Also known as infectious asthma.

ionizing radiation High-energy electromagnetic waves such as x-rays.

ischemia Deficiency of blood supply.

J

Jacksonian seizure A simple partial (focal or localized) seizure.

K

ketones Normal metabolic products from which acetone may arise spontaneously.

L

laryngectomy Excision of the larynx.

latex allergy A medical term encompassing a range of allergic reactions to natural rubber latex.

lumen The cavity of a tubular organ such as a blood vessel.

M

macrovascular disease Disease of the large vessels of the body.

mandible Lower jaw.

medical history Information obtained from a patient about past medical problems and medications that is useful in providing care to the patient.

microvascular disease Disease of the small vessels of the body.

myocardial infarction Circulatory emergency caused by occlusion of at least one of the coronary arteries.

myocardium Middle layer of the heart wall.

N

nasal cannula An attachment that can be used with the oxygen tank; the cannula fits into the patient's nostrils and delivers the oxygen.

negligence The omission of duty that results in injury or harm to another person.

neuropathy A nerve disorder that can cause numbness and sometimes pain and weakness in hands, arms, feet, and legs.

nitroglycerin A coronary vasodilator frequently prescribed for the prevention or relief of angina.

nonpsychogenic Physical, nonpsychological causes of a condition.

O

oral hypoglycemics Medication that can lower blood sugar.

orthostatic hypotension Decrease in blood pressure when a person is raised supine to erect.

oxygen tank A cylinder that contains oxygen.

P

pancreas Body organ that produces insulin.

partial (focal or localized) seizure Convulsive movements associated with epilepsy occurring on one side of the body only.

pericardium Sac that encloses the heart.

periodontal disease Disease of the periodontium.

personal protective equipment (PPE) Protective clothing and equipment, such as face shields and gloves, used in occupations to protect workers from injury and infection.

Physician's Desk Reference (PDR) Published book that provides information on various drugs.

presyncope First stage of syncope; stage prior to the actual loss of consciousness.

protected health information (PHI) Under the Health Insurance Portability and Accountability Act (HIPAA), any information about health status, provision of health care, or payment for health care that can be linked to a specific individual.

psychogenic Psychological causes of a condition.

pulmonary artery Artery that runs from the right ventricle to the lungs.

pulse The regular expansion and contraction of an artery caused by the ejection of the blood from the left ventricle of the heart as it contracts.

R

radial artery An artery located in the forearm.

regulator Attachment on an oxygen tank that allows oxygen to be released from the tank to the face mask or nasal cannula.

rescue breathing The act of assisting or stimulating respiration for a patient who is not breathing independently.

respiration rate The number of times that a person inhales and exhales.

S

semilunar valves A valve with half-moon-shaped cusps like the aortic valve and the pulmonary valve.

shock A life-threatening condition that occurs when the body is not getting enough blood flow.

sphygmomanometer Instrument that consists of a gauge and an inflatable bag inside an armband; used to measure blood pressure.

status asthmaticus A severe form of asthma in which the victim experiences a continuous asthma attack.

status epilepticus Situation in which a person experiences one seizure after another or one continuous seizure.

sternum Narrow, flat bone located at the midline of the thorax.

stethoscope Instrument used to listen to the heart and chest sounds.

stoma A small opening.

supine position Lying horizontally on the back.

syncope Fainting.

systolic pressure Pressure on the arteries when the heart is beating, or working.

T

temperature The level of heat in the body.

thrombosis A clot that forms in a vessel.

tonic Movements characterized by continuous tension or contraction of muscles that are associated with a tonic-clonic (grand mal) seizure.

tonic-clonic (grand mal) seizure An epileptic seizure characterized by generalized involuntary muscular contraction and cessation of respiration followed by tonic and clonic spasms of the muscles.

trachea The air passage that descends from the larynx and branches into the right and left bronchi; also known as the *windpipe*.

tracheobronchial tree The trachea, bronchi, and the bronchial tubes.

tracheotomy Incision made through the skin into the trachea to relieve an airway obstruction.

Trendelenburg position Position in which the patient is supine with the feet higher than the head.

U

universal precautions Approaches and protocols adopted to protect health care workers and their patients from getting and spreading disease and infection.

urticaria A skin reaction characterized by the eruption of itching wheals; also known as *hives*.

V

vasodilator An agent that causes the dilation of blood vessels.

ventricles Lower chambers of the heart.

vesicle An elevation of the epidermis containing fluid; also known as a *blister*.

X

xiphoid process Lowest portion of the sternum.

References

Publications

Bennett, J. D., & Rosenberg, M. B. (2002). *Medical emergencies in dentistry.* Philadelphia: W. B. Saunders.

Grimes, E. B. (2009). *Medical emergencies: Essentials for the dental professional.* Upper Saddle River, NJ: Pearson Prentice Hall.

Haas, D. A. (2010). Preparing dental office staff members for emergencies: Developing a basic action plan. *Journal of the American Dental Association.* Retrieved from http://jada.ada.org/content/141/suppl_1/8S.abstract

Little, J. W., Falace, D. Q., Miller, C. S., & Rhodus, N. L. (2002). *Dental management of the medically compromised patient* (6th ed.). St. Louis, MO: W. B. Saunders.

Malamed, S. F. (2007). *Medical emergencies in the dental office* (6th ed.). St. Louis, MO: Elsevier Health Sciences.

Phinney, D. J., & Halstead, J. H. (2008). *Dental assisting: A comprehensive approach* (3rd ed.). Clifton Park, NY: Thomson Learning/Delmar.

Pickett, F., & Guerenlian, J. (2005). *The medical history: Clinical implications and emergency prevention in dental settings.* Baltimore: Lippincott Williams & Wilkins.

Wilkins, E. M. (2005). *Clinical practice of the dental hygienist* (9th ed.). Baltimore: Lippincott Williams & Wilkins.

Internet Resources

American Dental Association, **http://www.ada.org**

American Diabetes Association, **http://www.diabetes.org**

American Heart Association, **http://www.heart.org/HEARTORG**

American Heart Association, 2010 Guidelines for Cardiopulmonary Resuscitation and Emergency Cardiovascular Care, **http://guidelines.ecc.org/2010-guidelines -for-cpr.html**

American Lung Association, **http://www.lungusa.org**

American Red Cross, **http://www.redcross.org**

American Stroke Association, **http://www.strokeassociation.org/STROKEORG**

Epilepsy Foundation, **http://epilepsyfoundation.org**

Index